Midwifery
is catching

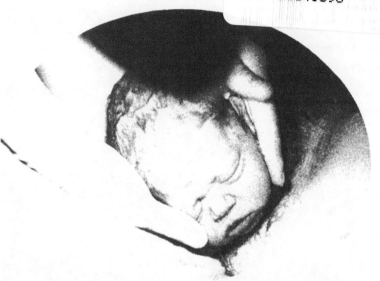

According to midwifery philosophy, credit for "delivering" a baby belongs to the mother. Her midwife is there to aid and abet, and then to gently "catch" the arriving infant.

This book is dedicated to my courageous Mom, who taught us all to question and speak out.

And to dear Dad, quiet spirit of optimism.

with love,
Ellie

"I've had seven children, in three hospitals, in three Canadian cities, and I hope that none of you girls ever has to go through what I went through."
Patricia Barrington R.N.
circa 1970

Midwifery
is catching

Eleanor Barrington

NC Press Limited
Toronto, 1985

Canadian Cataloguing in Publication Data
Barrington, Eleanor, 1956-
   Midwifery is catching
Bibliography: p.
ISBN 0-920053-35-1
1. Midwives – Canada.   2. Childbirth – Canada.
3. Obstetrics – Canada.
I. Title
RG950.B37 1985   618.2'0233   C85-098375-4

We would like to thank the Ontario Arts Council and the Canada Council for their assistance in the production of this book.

Cover Photography, Bill Usher
Cover Design, Rob Finnemore
Typesetting, Jay Tee Graphics Ltd.
Printing and Binding, Hignell Printing Ltd.

New Canada Publications, a division of NC Press Limited,
Box 4010 Station A, Toronto, Ontario M5H 1H8

Contents

A Personal Preface

I believe that childbirth is mostly safe and always sacred. I view it as a natural challenge to be met rather than an ordeal to be avoided. These are not accepted convictions about birth in Canadian culture, but then my initiation to birthing was rather unorthodox.

The first child I saw born arrived with the dawning light in her mother's living room. A sensitive midwife oversaw Iselina's journey from womb to world. The child was enveloped in the tearful welcome of a room full of women, and loving hands carried her immediately to her mother's breast.

Her mother Christine had laboured only five hours for this first child. A study in concentration, she channeled her energy with deep sighs down through her overbloomed belly, smoothing through the pain of each contraction.

Iselina's birth was not an event too holy for humour, nor too magical to admit the midwife's medical precautions. But its essence was reverence. Reverence for both mother and child. They governed the progress of the birthing. They experienced its completion in uninterrupted bonding.

Other home births with various midwives followed. Some were likewise spiritually streamlined, some animal practical, some rather more medically complex. Each was a blueprint for an emerging personality, a reflection of the lives and psyches of the becoming parents.

My attitudes to birth began to crystallize. I realized that to be true to my research, I had to see what birth looked like to other people. Most Canadians go to hospital without a midwife.

I had heard a hundred intimate hospital horror stories by then. In search of balance, I read the literature about birth reform in our institutions: family-centred care, natural childbirth, birthing rooms, respect for bonding.

Tallying the effect of my favourable experience of midwife-attended home births, I truly expected to be influenced by the progressive advances at a downtown Toronto teaching hospital. I suspected that my critical picture of the hospital-medical birth model would fill in with the mid-tones of wise compromise. Many mothers, after all, are quite satisfied with their doctor-in-hospital births.

I arrived at the hospital in excited anticipation, as always, at the prospect of birth. I observed incognito.

Perhaps it was a bad day, although it wasn't busy. Perhaps it was bad luck, or the negative preconceptions I tried to leave behind. But what I saw was my personal version of Orwell's *1984*.

Newspeak: The catch words of the birthing movement bandied about, while actions spoke the opposite. "Natural childbirth" with epidurals and episiotomies? "Bonding" when mother and baby never touch? A nurse intones mechanically while she counts sterile swabs: "Now you relax. You just relax and breathe." Is this labour support hospital-style?

"No. I won't give you any medication," the anaesthetist assures a woman about to have twins as he inserts a spinal shunt, just in case she needs an epidural for an emergency cesarean. "I'll put in just enough to test that the anaesthetic will go through." Meanwhile he pours out a substantial 6 cc dose. "No. It won't get to the baby," he lies outright to the enquiring father.

That non-epidural ends the mother's healthy contractions for a full two hours, postponing the birth of her twins. Luckily, her doctor is willing to wait.

In the course of three labours and births that day I silently watch uncomfortable fathers, distanced from their mates by the sterile environment, unsure of where to stand or whether they could touch their wives. I saw four infants enter the world through the gaping blood baths of routine episiotomies, only to be whisked away from their mothers. Exiled to sterile heating tables, they screamed out their shock at an untouching world. Meanwhile, mother's eyes silently swept the delivery room in search of the child of her labour.

These were random births, anybody births. One Laotian couple irritated their nurse by not speaking English. They couldn't understand the epidural she was offering. An epidural this particular mother clearly did not need. When she finally comprehended and consented, the nurse decided she couldn't have it after all.

One couple was quite pleased with their second birth. "Epidural is the best thing ever invented," declared the mother as they took her baby away.

One well-researched couple travelled a long way for a natural twin birth after a cesarean. They were allowed vaginal birth, if not a natural one. But the mother didn't get to hold those fat, healthy babies. Her determination was not defense enough against hospital routine.

I returned from those births exhausted rather than exhilarated, so I was glad when my research offered me a reassuringly positive experience of hospital birth. The nurse who allowed me into the birthing room along with Wendee and Peter and midwife Jane (see chapter five), did more good than she knew. Clearly hospitals could serve parents' best interests, if they had the knowledgeable support of a midwife.

My own first pregnancy progressed along with the writing of this book, making the work and the words immediate and real. With the support of our doctors and midwives, my husband Steven and I made the very personal choice to plan for a home birth — with alternate hospital arrangements.

I went into labour once the book was safely packaged for the publisher. Yet it was a full week after my son Liam was born before I realized *why* I had written it. Indeed, why, as a single woman without children, had I been drawn to this issue back in 1981?

Because I was going to really *need* my midwives. And so would Liam, to have the kind of birth he deserved.

My labour was an arduous 24 hours. Nothing romantic about those hours of pain with no apparent progress. I wouldn't have had the courage to refuse painkilling drugs if they had been handy. In hospital, even my non-interventive doctor would have felt pressure to *do* something. Labour had begun with my waters breaking, thus imposing a medical deadline. There is a good chance that Liam and I would have joined the cesarean section statistics, in spite of all my convictions about natural birth.

But my midwives Theo and Mary did not find my peculiar course of progress abnormal. They simple responded to my unspoken needs, intuiting that pressure would help here, pillows there. Steven took their cues in coming to my aid. Sometimes I needed absolute silence, sometimes constant verbal direction. They transformed furniture into comfortable props for different labouring positions. All the while, the midwives' reports reminded me that whatever I was enduring, my baby was faring extremely well. That helped.

Eventually I reached a point where I cried that I couldn't stand it anymore. And perhaps *because* I couldn't stand it, I finally pushed myself to face the pain. I began to concentrate on the waves of each contraction, chanting to myself: "Sweet pain. Baby pain." And it worked! Not that the pain went away, but the more I concentrated, the better I coped. Theo, fingers at my cervix, reported that it was now rapidly softening and opening. My arms and legs no longer tensed against each rising wave. My body went limp and all my energy stayed in my uterus.

Sensing that I needed neither outside help nor distraction now, Mary and Theo banked me up on pillows and left me in the dark with Steven as watch. Within one hour I progressed from six to ten centimetres and through transition to pushing — all in peaceful silence. Shortly thereafter, Mary caught Liam and I reached out to bring him to my breast. Oh, wonder!

The immediate pay-off for my hard labour was Liam's vibrant good health. He was born breathing, pink to the toes, alert. He wasn't drugged and he was met by tender hands. My son didn't bother to cry, preferring to suck instead. Liam has remained a calm, if actively demanding, infant.

His birth brought me a personal windfall as well. I discovered my own powers of concentration, healing and meditation. I might never have otherwise put myself to a test that has won me great confidence. Now I understand why women are so strong. A standard medical birth would probably have denied me that knowledge.

In the week following Liam's birth, I began to perceive a flaw in my book. It does not pay enough attention to the midwife's role during the postpartum roller coaster of ecstasy and exhaustion. Theo, Mary and our good Dr. Harris answered hundreds of naive questions. We anxiously awaited their daily visits, bringing advice and solace to calm our new-parent angst. And at 6 a.m. on Sunday morning, when your screaming baby cannot seem to latch onto your overfull breast, a midwife's phone number is a prize without price!

When I set out to write this book, I thought I was doing it for other families. I felt that people deserved better care and more caring than they were getting; that babies deserved better beginnings. I wanted to spread the good news that midwifery was happening again in this country, that there was a viable alternative to hospital birth and a more satisfying way to give birth in hospital as well. But I know now that I researched and wrote this book for myself and my family. I hope that it helps you to find what you need too.

— Eleanor Barrington, November 1984

Chapter One
Better Care, More Caring

Upstairs:

Diane and Chris work together and their labour day moves along. Midwives Mary Sharpe and Catherine Penz support Diane's limbs as she moves once again onto hands and knees. They observe silently while she calls out the long deep note of her labour song, uttered rhythmically during this and every contraction. Then they gently instruct Chris on how to use his weight to relieve the pressure of his wife's painful back labour.

Diane's concentration is directed inward. She expresses herself in blind trust to her birthing team. At times she is a wise lady of seventy, at other moments a whining seven-year-old. She is accomplishing birth in her own unique way, on her own time.

An event-free daylight first stage gears up to two hours of determined pushing at suppertime. Finally, a dark-haired scalp appears and a midwife guides Diane's hand down to touch her baby. The room explodes with the joy of this first mother-child meeting. Diane renews her pushes with the energy of love and adrenalin.

The baby's head stretches at Diane's perineum. Mary applies hot compresses and coaxes the opening with olive oil and perineal massage. The midwives pace Diane's breathing to ease the baby out slowly, while Mary sets one tiny ear free, and then the other. Catherine is poised to suction mucous from mouth and nose as the baby's head is born. Cradling his wife in his arms, Chris watches transfixed in a mirror someone holds up for him.

With knowing hands, Mary guides the shoulders over an intact perineum. Then she leads Diane's hands down to her half-born child. Mother draws her son out of her own body and up onto her breast. Chris enfolds them both. The birth is complete. The family is born. The atmosphere is euphoria.

Downstairs:

Chris' mother paces uneasy. She expresses her admiration for the birthstyle going on upstairs, but is unable to really trust it. Over 60, self-declared feminist, the kind of grande dame who loses her husband and proceeds to go back to university with her son, Madeleine tries to be rational about her overflowing emotions. But when she visits the birthing room for a few contractions she bursts into tears and retreats. Not just empathy, she admits, but also memory.

Her experiences of birth were very unhappy. Decades later, she realizes that the emotional pain of childbirth is still with her. *She* never had the tender caresses her Chris offers Diane. She never had the constant support of midwives. She was alone and fearful. It was an ordeal, she explains, discreetly dabbing her tears.

Madeleine is overjoyed when the baby is safely born. She jokes to Diane that she, too, has had a hard labour today. This birth, with the midwives, is the better way, she confirms. She is proud of Diane's courage, and perhaps a little suprised to have learned faith in birth from her daughter-in-law.

— Toronto, January 1984

*   *   *

What a curious moment in Canadian childbirth culture, that mothers should be learning about birth from their daughters! It is not an uncommon experience in the 1980s. So many of our mothers, deprived of consciousness, of personal support, of the very physical experience of birth, look on in awe and admiration while we plan our natural births. At first they think us naive or crazy. Then they wonder what they missed.

It is no coincidence that the generations deprived of their childbirth experiences were the same generations who missed out on the midwives. It was the advance of medical science, the monopoly of doctor-care, and the supposed safety of hospital birth that created the sociological deviation that was childbirth in our mothers' time. The midwives, along with our mothers, were sacrificed to progress. While midwives' practices were far from perfect, the real reason the wise women disappeared was that they stood for something different: they believed in women giving birth.

During the early decades of this century, the tradition of community midwifery in Canada was virtually wiped out by the advancing medical profession. Two or three generations gave birth without any option of midwifery care. They gave up childbirth to the doctor, in the name of pain relief and safety, or simply because they had no choice.

New Midwives in Canada

The sweep of social change in the 1960s sowed the seeds of many new ideas across Canada, and unearthed some old ones. The long-dormant community tree of midwifery was grafted with a new attitude to birth, so that a hybrid they called "the new midwifery" bloomed in the early seventies.

A vanguard of young parents began seeking a more fulfilling experience of birth than the medical system could offer. Their motivations could be described as enlightened self-interest or evolving consciousness, but what they wanted was clear. They acknowledged the creative complexity of childbirth, and they chose to protect and enhance it as a natural process.

The first "new midwives" emerged from among these questioning parents. Mothers who explored and experimented first for themselves, shared their newfound skills and experience with their neighbours. They gave birth at home, and whoever knew more offered help. Most were reticent to accept the title of midwife until it was thrust upon them by others.

Unlike the granny midwives of earlier generations, these new midwives were not handed an intact tradition. They redefined midwifery through their work and research, according to the needs and norms of their particular communities.

The hybrid midwifery practices that evolved in the 1970s were inevitably mixtures of old art, modern science and new age insight. Resourceful midwives borrowed herbs and old wives tales from native and ethnic midwifery practices. They spent hours palpating blooming bellies to develop the sensitive diagnostic touch that has always been a midwife's essential tool. They learned from elderly "granny midwives" wherever they could find them, and then they turned to the obstetrical texts. In the first years, the training of a midwife was entirely self-directed and self-motivated. Everyone entered practice via a different path.

In pursuit of safety, midwives sought sympathetic physicians to provide adequate emergency back-up. Many found general practitioners willing to share their knowledge of birth complications and emergency management.

True to their community roots, some midwives swear by herbs, and others carry ultrasound. But over the years, standards of practice, if not styles, have become more uniform across the country.

Since the first midwives appeared in British Columbia in 1972, perhaps 200 women have accepted the onerous responsibilities and joyous rewards of midwifery without benefit of legal status in Canada. Thousands of Canadian couples have received support and service throughout their reproductive cycle that most others dare not dream of.

Several thousand Canadian babies have been safely ushered into this world and tenderly caught by the midwives. These families have experienced a standard of maternity care that the medical delivery system simply cannot offer.

In the early years of midwifery activity, the secret of their services was passed in cautious whispers to close friends. Nowadays, word about the midwives is announced in the national media. With an expanding power base of satisfied parents and concerned health professionals, more and more Canadian midwives are coming out of the closet. The midwifery movement, a tiny birthing minority, is having a disproportionately large public opinion impact.

In a society where individuals increasingly dare to demand the best for themselves, midwifery offers better care, and more caring, than the medical maternity system. As evidence of the superior safety of midwifery finally reaches public light, it is no wonder that midwifery is catching on.

What is a Midwife?

Canada is unique among Western industrialized countries in having no midwifery system. Of all the 210 member countries of the World Health Organization, we share this dubious distinction with only eight third world states: Venezuela, Panama, New Hebrides, Honduras, El Salvador, Dominican Republic, Columbia and Berundi. Thus re-introducing midwifery to Canadians begins with the task of definition. In Canada, (and only in Canada — pity!) one hears the innocent question: "What is a midwife?"

"Mid-wife" is an Old English derivation meaning "with the woman." In the French culture, she is a "sage-femme," their wise woman. Today's midwife is by turns friend and neighbour, doctor and nurse, teacher and therapist, grandmother and priest. She is a domestic helper, a community worker, and a feminist health activist. Chances are, she is also someone's mother and someone's sweetheart. A midwife doesn't get much sleep!

The definition of midwifery adopted by many of the birthing support organizations in Canada is the one developed by the International Confederation of Midwives and the International Federation of Gynecology and Obstetrics. It is used by the World Health Organization.

> A midwife is a person who, having been regularly admitted to a midwifery educational programme, duly recognised in the country in which it is located, has successfully completed the prescribed course of studies in midwifery and has acquired the requisite qualifications to be registered and/or legally licensed to practise midwifery.

She must be able to give the necessary supervision, care and advice to women during pregnancy, labour, and the post-partum period, to conduct deliveries on her own responsibility and to care for the newborn and infant. This care includes preventative measures, the detection of abnormal conditions in mother and child, the procurement of medical assistance and the execution of emergency measures in the absence of medical help.

She has an important task in health counselling and education not only for patients but also within the family and community. The work should involve ante-natal education and preparation for parenthood and extends to certain areas of gynaecology, family planning and child care.[1]

Since there is no school of midwifery duly recognized in Canada, our midwives cannot acquire the requisite qualifications formally. But most active midwives aspire to this definition, and many fulfill it in other jurisdictions.

Myths and Misconceptions

The Canadian midwife, with her interrupted heritage, must define herself against a background of myths and misconceptions, some of which have thoroughly permeated public opinion. Dorothy Hall, former Director of Nursing Education for the World Health Organization, quoted in the *Kitchener-Waterloo Record*, recalls leaving Canada for Asia in the 1940s, "believing that midwifery was a medieval practice that should be wiped out." Her international experience rapidly reversed that thinking.

Such impressions had their beginnings in the 16th-century witchhunt of women healers, and were furthered by the 20th-century campaign against North American midwives. This latter offensive, manned by the medical profession, characterized the Canadian midwife as a slovenly, ignorant old granny with dirty hands.

No doubt a few were. Jutta Mason's as yet unpublished research unearthed Dr. Kendal's *Early Medical Experiences In Cape Breton Island*. In it we meet a granny midwife "somewhat the worse for gin. . .smoking a blackened clay pipe. . .thumping the table and roaring with laughter" while the young physician boiled his instruments in a potato pot. Yet one can't help but wonder if Dr. Kendal was really any more useful than the drunken granny, at what he admits was his "first accouchement."

Studies demonstrating midwives' birth outcomes to be at least as good as doctors in the early decades of the century were suppressed.[2] Instead, the slovenly granny was so thoroughly promoted that she might have blackened the midwife's image forever, were it not for the sterling reputation of another sort of midwife. Aunt Lucy of Labrador is her embodiment:

> Aunt Lucy [is the] mother and aunt to two villages, over 60 years old, who travelled night and day over roads, waded through mud, slush and slob, clung to boats and wallowed through snow to get to some expectant mother. Then she would sit up 12 or 24 hours waiting for the baby. . . .She was the mainstay of the community.
> — from *Nurse Banfield in Labrador*

Current midwives can make jokes about their brooms. They laugh along with embarrassed women who call expecting any midwife to be as old as grandma. What they find more upsetting are the recent misconceptions, promulgated by some uninformed physicians. Sometimes midwives are described as glorified labour coaches, who do little more than help a woman breathe. One Toronto obstetrician disparaged them as "uneducated women playing backroom doctor."

A "hippy midwife" caricature, put forward on the basis of the new midwifery's early beginnings, relegates the midwife's work to an outdated fringe of society. In fact, by 1980, the majority of midwives and their clients belonged to the middle class. Today's "wise woman" is likely to be about thirty-five, raised in a suburb, and university educated. If she wears her hair long and her skirts flowing, that is her personal style. She feels no need to don a white coat to assert her professionalism.

The concept of "spiritual midwifery," popularized by the book of that title, has been a source of much honest confusion. The spiritual midwife works with birth as part of the ebb and flow of life, acknowledging forces beyond the physical process. But she is not a witch doctor who merely voices incantations when action is required.

The midwifery of "The Farm" community in Tennessee described in *Spiritual Midwifery* boasts some of the best perinatal outcome statistics in the United States. After ten years and 1,200 high- and low-risk births,[3] this good record cannot be attributed to luck, or even divine intercession. Their spirituality provides a context, *not* a substitute, for knowledge and technique. The most "spiritual" of the midwives study obstetrical texts.

A further misconception which complicates many midwives' images, is a confusion about the distinctions between nursing and midwifery. It arises because thousands of so-called nurse-midwives, trained in other countries, populate our obstetrical wards. Women who are both nurses and midwives are reduced to the former role in Canadian hospitals.

Nursing is not considered internationally to be a prerequisite for midwifery training although there is some use of nursing skills in midwifery practice. Some midwives are nurses first. Many are not.

The final myth to be exposed is the popular equation of midwifery and home birth, two very separate concerns. The coupling of these two issues has occurred in Canada because midwives have no status in the hospital system. Many midwives are only able to do their work in the domicilliary setting. But wherever hospital policy permits them entry, the new midwives offer all of their services — short of baby catching — to families that prefer the hospital birth venue. In hospitals their actions are curtailed, but they can act as parent advocates.

Internationally, midwives enjoy a status like doctors, and can attend births in hospitals, birth centres or homes. The new midwives in Canada have voiced their desire to serve birthing women in their venue of choice. Most Canadians, it is assumed, will continue to prefer a hospital, or a birth centre, when that option becomes available.

The Midwifery Care Model

The *personality* or style of a midwife's practice comes from the community she serves, be it outport or hamlet or urban metropolis. Geographic, cultural and social factors define the ways in which midwives work, because they and their services grow out of the community. But there is a distinctive model of care which can be uncovered in almost any new midwife's practice. All adhere to a set of philosophical and practical tenets that make them midwives.

By international recognition, the midwife is the specialist in normal birth. Her training focuses on the healthy process of parturition, and how to facilitate this process without upsetting nature's intricate balance.

The midwife's concept of normal birth sometimes differs from current medical definition. It includes a broad range of possibilities — and time frames — indicative of individual mothers' personalities and processes. Having watched births proceed to healthy conclusions without interventions in the home setting, many midwives refuse to be bound by certain medical standards of normalcy. The Friedman Curve, for instance, sets out the medically acceptable length of time for the stages of normal labour and delivery. The first-time mother is allowed two hours between full dilation and delivery, the multip only one. Some women and some babies, the midwives assert, quite normally take longer. One midwife laughs that she has never seen a normal birth. The standard woman it presumes just doesn't exist!

Midwives are also, of course, able to screen for high risk pregnancies, recognize complications, and manage emergencies. In such cases, they call in medical expertise. The obstetrician is the specialist in abnormal birth. He has studied for years what can go wrong, and how to cope with it.

But her role does not end with the detection of complications. Holistic care and continuous support are perhaps more vital to the high risk mother and child. A midwife works in concert with the obstetrician, hoping to minimize or eliminate risks. In Sweden virtually every woman, low or high risk, has a midwife. The birth outcome statistics support this policy.

By definition a specialist in normal birth, the new midwife has also become the guardian of natural birth, when that is the preference of her client. A truly natural birth is not desirable or appropriate for every woman, but it is the standard toward which a midwife works. She seeks to limit intervention in the normal physical and psychological process, to a degree appropriate for the individual woman. She also sets a standard for defining ''natural'' childbirth, of late a much misused catchphrase. As Barbara Katz Rothman points out in her book *In Labour:* ''Natural childbirth is a slippery concept: it may mean anything from there being no surgical incision at the time of the birth. . .to consciousness alone, even with an epidural or spinal anaesthetic.''[4]

Natural childbirth means birth without medical interference, not labour pain without relief. While a woman's body is governing the progress of her normal labour, a midwife offers non-interventive pain relief, and to some extent, pain prevention. She provides information which reduces fear, and her constant presence alleviates the loneliness and insecurity that creates tension in so many mothers. Physical comforts like massage, touching, and compresses are potent painkillers. Eye contact, verbal encouragement, and suggestions that a woman change positions from time to time, are also among the aids a midwife employs.

Midwives work to reinforce a woman's confidence in her body's capability. They attempt to open a pregnant woman up to her own innate knowledge about birth, because she alone can deliver her baby. Birth, according to the midwifery philosophy, is an accomplishment exclusive to mothers. Midwives can only catch the babies delivered by moms.

The key to many of the basic tenets of midwifery is *care*, and it is the nature of that care that makes midwifery so safe. Of all the countries in the World Health Organization, those with the most developed midwifery systems consistently rank highest in comparisons of birth outcomes. That is because of continuous care, preventative care, holistic care, and individualized, family-centred care.

Continuous care extends right through the reproductive cycle and into early parenting. (Perhaps through several cycles.) It includes constant support and monitoring by one individual throughout labour and delivery.

Continuous care, involving generous commitments of time, allows a midwife to gather a store of impressions that will substantiate future intuitions and actions. Her familiarity with the norms of mother and babe enables her to notice deviations from those norms immediately.

Her vigilant presence during labour may be vital to detect physical warning signals, but it also affects the psychological determinants in birth. Emotional upsets manifest in physical complications. Studies have shown that any animal, if frightened during labour, will cease its contractions until it finds a place of safety.[5] The human female is equally vulnerable. Research has demonstrated that the presence of a supportive lay woman throughout labour shortens its duration and reduces perinatal problems.[6]

The preventative focus of midwifery includes such factors as nutrition, exercise, rest, and emotional stress. It involves support for lifestyle changes — quitting smoking, avoiding alcohol, etc. — that might otherwise have deleterious effects on the baby. Midwives provide a therapeutic listening environment for mothers and partners to work through the difficult transitions into parenthood.

A preventative approach cuts many potential physical complications off at the pass. For example, a nutritional shift at five months might avoid a prematurely induced labour for pre-eclampsia at eight.

The holism in midwifery refers to the whole woman, for her whole reproductive cycle, in her whole environment. A pregnant woman is a physical, emotional and social being, and none of these factors can be safely ignored. Similarly, no one event in her reproductive cycle can be adequately analyzed without reference to what has come before.

A midwife's advice must be tailored to the real circumstances of her client's life. There is little sense in telling the woman who *has* to work until her due date that she ought to be sleeping in the afternoons. Better to suggest she put her feet up for a few minutes at lunch. While quitting smoking altogether would be the preferred action for any pregnant woman, a wise midwife will assess the daily hurdles her client has to overcome, and then decide what kind of cigarette reduction to ask for. She steers her clients off disastrous paths, and looks for signs of individual progress.

Family-centred care acknowledges that whatever is happening in the family (or the co-op, or a single mother's support circle) has repercussions for mother and child. Everyone in a household is affected by a new baby, and often, everyone wants to feel involved. Often the midwife's job includes counselling for a new father, or birth education for young siblings. Couples attend prenatal visits together, often with a curious toddler in tow. When it suits the parents' wishes, this culminates with the whole family present at the birth.

Midwifery care involves a partnership in responsibility with parents. Acknowledging that *they* will live with the consequences, parents are encouraged to make their own, well-informed birthing decisions. Especially in the current legal climate, a midwife cannot encourage parents to abdicate their power and authority. She provides information, advice, experience and skills, and helps them to find birthing satisfaction. But parents must make their own decisions.

Once they have made choices of attendant, of venue and of birthstyle, she supports them. A midwife often becomes mediator between conscious parents and a not-so-conscious public. Her goal is to steer each couple toward *their* best possible birth.

The Medical Care Gap

For several decades medicine had a monopoly on maternity care in Canada. With no competition, and no comparison, it was generally accepted as the only safe way to have a child.

Recently, people have been discovering that in other places, and under different care systems, some parents have it better. The consumer movement has made information about alternatives readily available, and the midwifery movement provides a model for comparison. Seeing it, many parents are unwilling to accept less.

No one would denigrate the contribution of modern medicine to the improved physical safety of the high risk mother and child. In this field, the doctors have made persistent progress for the last few decades. Babies, and mothers, who would once have died are now surviving.

However, in focussing heroic efforts on the perhaps impossible task of eliminating death from birth, the obstetrical profession has narrowed its vision. Seeing only the physical risks of childbirth, it has lost sight of the psychological and social aspects which are inextricably linked to physical outcomes. Searching always for what might go wrong, even in a normal pregnancy and birth, the obstetrical profession has clearly lost faith in nature's process.

Modern obstetrics clouds birth with a disfiguring fear, instead of enhancing it with a visionary confidence. Mounting scientific evidence indicts obstetrical practice for creating birth complications. Intervening out of impatience or fear, much obstetrical activity upsets the natural progress of otherwise uncomplicated births. The belief that birth is a crisis clearly creates crises.

The biggest hole in the medical maternity model is a lack of continuity and time. It is simply not economical for even the most dedicated doctor to provide adequate hours for preventative prenatal care. Nor can he afford to sit through entire labours, often inactive. Thus the services needed by birthing women are divided up piecemeal in the medical delivery system, or not offered at all.

In the course of standard medical maternity care, one woman might see her family doctor, an obstetrician, several labour and delivery nurses, an intern or obstetrical resident, an anaesthetist, her obstetrician's call partner, a postpartum nurse, a pediatrician, a family planning representative and a public health nurse. One familiar midwife could replace half the parade of new faces, and provide a vital communication link between those personnel still required. As a continuous presence, she would be best informed about the particular birth.

The practice of leaving labouring women entirely alone is all but unique to North America in this century. Because of the division of labour among hospital staff, a nurse (or several of them) makes sporadic checks of the vital signs. This does not qualify as birth support by any standard. Nor is it truly safe. The recent admission of nervous and ill-equipped fathers into the labour rooms has done little to alleviate the actual care-gap. Social anthropologists point out that even among primitive tribes, our custom would be pronounced barbaric.[7] Such is the lonely heart of Canadian childbirth culture.

The Canadian Medical Association reports an 85% male medical profession in Canada in 1984. Thus we have a major gender gap in maternity care. Modern obstetrics is condemned by feminist analysis of the oppression and abuse of what is innately female. Birthing women are increasingly concerned about ending decades of male dominance over their bodies. They want women in support as their maternity care givers, not men in charge.

As well as the safety gap (to be discussed more fully in Chapter Eight) and the sociological gaps, there is a major service gap between the medical system and the birth movement. Accustomed to a comfortable monopoly for so long, the medical care delivery system is slow to offer real choices and alternatives. "Progressive" hospitals now pay lip service to natural childbirth and family-centred care. Close scrutiny usually reveals these innovations to be co-optations of the demands of the public.

This gap is the catalyst that has propelled the midwifery movement into the public eye in the 1980s. Canadians are service-conscious consumers. A middle-class couple can afford the time and energy to shop around, and now has the confidence to demand the best. They want information, choices and personalized attention. Rarely does a doctor have the time or inclination to provide all this. A midwife offers the kind of available care, and caring, women want for themselves, and at a very reasonable cost. Once young couples are aware of the midwifery option, most are unwilling to settle for less.

Midwifery will never replace medical maternity care. High risk mothers need all the benefits of modern obstetrics as well as midwifery care. Midwives need emergency medical back-up. And many couples simply prefer to stay with their familiar family doctors. What Canadian women deserve, and what they will fight to get during the '80s, is universal access to a *choice* of caregivers; to midwifery and obstetrics as complementary services.

Our Changing Childbirth Culture

> The act of giving birth to a child is never simply a physical act, but rather a performance, defined by and enacted within a cultural context.[8]
>
> — Shelley Romalis

Midwifery has had a cultural impact far in excess of the minority who have personally experienced a midwife's care. It has promoted a new definition and context for birth. Because this alternative vision is in the air, many parents' expectations and involvement has increased. People dare to demand more of themselves and their doctors.

The presence of midwives has affected hospital personnel and policy. Observing the midwife's effectiveness up close, obstetrical nurses, residents and physicians are often provoked to adapt their own actions and attitudes. As the mainstream system slowly begins to change, the performance of birth is allowed more creative leeway.

Unlike some of the birth movements that came before, midwifery has not only increased consumer awareness and expectations, it has provided a means for realizing those expectations. Consequently childbirth in our culture is visibly changing. Ideas that once belonged to the counter-culture have moved into the middle-class mainstream. Giving birth is viewed by an increasing minority as a woman's opportunity to explore her own strength, and as a family opportunity to grow together.

Birth is taking on a dimension that our mothers cannot recognize. Women describe it as creative self-expression, even as a sensual experience, albeit accompanied by purposeful pain. There are now births that smell human instead of antiseptic. There are birth-days for the whole family, when the woman's cries may be cries of ecstacy rather than agony, and when the gently welcomed babe may not need to cry out at all.

Performed within this new cultural context, childbirth can indeed be as Sheila Kitzinger describes it: "A creative drama of Wagnerian magnitude." And that is what the new midwives stand for.

Notes

1. International Definition of Midwifery, International Federation of Gynaecology and Obstetrics and the International Confederation of Midwives, (FIGO/ICM), *Maternity Care in the World, Second Edition,* 1976, pp. x-xi.
2. Judy B. Litoff, *American Midwives: 1860 to the Present.*
3. Ina May Gaskin, *Spiritual Midwifery.*
4. Barbara Rothman, PhD, *In Labor: Women and Power in the Workplace,* p. 79.
5. Niles Newton, "The Effect of Fear and Disturbance on Labour" in *21 Century Obstetrics Now!* ed. Stewart & Stewart.
6. Roberto Sosa, M.D. et al, "The Effect of a Supportive Companion on Perinatal Problems, Length of Labor and Mother-Infant Interaction," *New England Journal of Medicine,* September 11, 1980.
7. Doris Haire, "The Cultural Warping of Childbirth," A Special Report, International Childbirth Education Association, 1972.
8. Shelley Romalis, *Childbirth Alternatives to Medical Control,* p. 6.

Mark Laforet

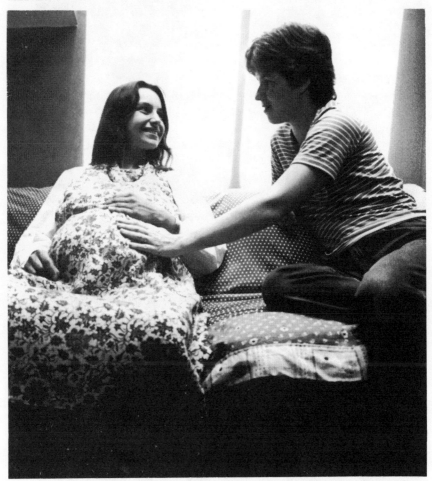

Midwife Gale Gray with hand on client's belly.

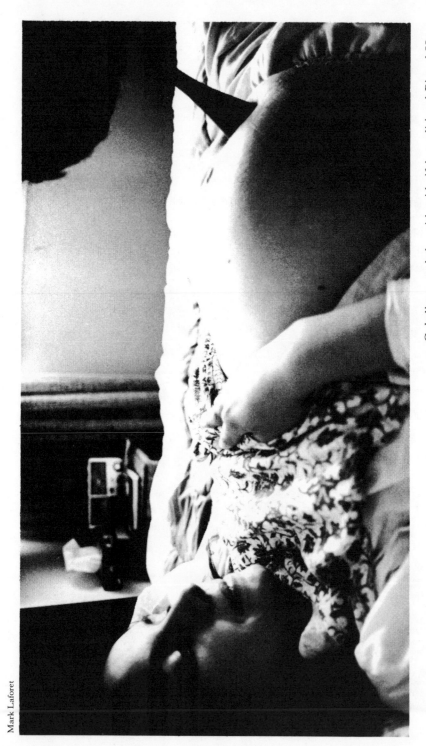

Mark Laforet

Gale listens to baby with midwife's traditional Pinard Horn.

Chapter Two
Decline and Renaissance

The women of Ville Marie, in solemn enclave assembled, on February 12, 1713, elected a midwife, Catherine Guertain, for the community. . . the first instance of votes for women having been employed in this province.[1]

— *Dr. Maude Abbott*

The community midwife was not always an elected official like Catherine Guertain of Montreal, but until the twentieth century, she remained an esteemed figure in most Canadian towns. The reluctant decline of community midwifery in Canada stretched over most of a century, and is attributed to the rise of a male-dominated medical profession after 1850.[2] The organization of the medical profession, legislation supporting the medical monopoly of health care, and the twentieth century trend toward hospital birth all contributed to the near demise of the Canadian midwife by the 1940s. Faced with organized upper-class men who had the law and science on their side, poor and often illiterate community midwives, isolated from one another, had little hope of retaining sway.

Midwifery History: Doctor versus Midwife

Until 1850, lay healers and midwives still abounded in all parts of Canada. Doctors took little or no interest in attending births. But during the 1850s, the growing number of doctors trying to make a living in Toronto and Montreal began to look to the accouchement as an entré to family practice. In Nova Scotia, which also had a relatively high physician population, doctors began to encroach on the midwife's territory in the 1860s. Elsewhere in the country, this advance was delayed for a decade or two.

In 1865, a statute of the Province of Canada placed midwifery under the jurisdiction of licensed medical practitioners.[3] It is an indication of the community midwife's popularity that this statute did not reflect actual practice for several decades. In the 1870s midwives still taught medical students their obstetrics at the University Lying In Hospital in Montreal and the Burnside Hospital in Toronto.[4]

When the newly-formed College of Physicians and Surgeons of Ontario began to focus on the prosecution of unlicensed practitioners after 1874, even *The Globe* newspaper came out in support of the midwives. An editorial of August 24, 1875 entitled ''Medicus On The Warpath,'' berated the College: "In no way does the restriction. . .operate more harshly and unreasonably than in imposing the terms of the law between women and the assistance they are accustomed to rely upon from members of their own sex."

In Ontario, as elsewhere, doctors were tolerant of the midwives until they developed an economic interest in birth. A letter to the medical journal *Canada Lancet* in 1873 admits that deliveries are "to many of us country doctors a very remunerative part of our practice," and regrets the loss of income to "old bodies and a quack."[5]

While this doctor charged five dollars, and a midwife charged only two, he did not likely offer a safer or superior service. Earlier doctors were advised to leave their forceps at home "lest the impatience of the patient, the anxiety of the friends, or the doctor's wish to show that he was really doing something" provoke their premature and dangerous use.[6] But by the 1880s the currently lamented trend toward medical intervention in childbirth was already underway. In 1885, *Canada Lancet* prophesied: "At the present rate of advance (in forceps use) we shall soon overtake Nature and relegate her to a back place."

The competition between doctors and midwives was played out on the home birth front for several decades, because only destitute and unwed mothers would submit to hospitalization during the last century. Hospitals were filthy, crowded, unventilated, and evidently members of the staff "took full advantage of the patients' brandy and whiskey allowance." Jo Oppenheimer writes that many patients died in epidemics in hospital, and people feared that they would be used for experimentation. In Ontario in 1899 only 789 babies were born in hospitals.

But she found that many mothers in Ontario, the most medically advanced province, were delivered by physicians at home. The example of Queen Victoria, and the urban upper classes from whose ranks the doctors were drawn, began to popularize "doctor-births." Only one-sixth of recorded births in Ontario were not attended by doctors by 1897 and few of those "medically unattended" births admitted to their midwives.[7]

Midwives rooted in community tradition elsewhere in the country retained influence well into this century. As late as 1924 New Brunswick and Saskatchewan doctors reported 50% medically unattended births in their provinces.[8]

In British Columbia community midwifery had never really gotten a widespread start. Outside of the Victorian Order of Nurses, B.C. was not settled until the turn of the century, after the long push through the Rocky Mountains. Mining company doctors, anxious to practice obstetrics from the start, arrived along with the population. Similarly in the Yukon, doctors came along with the gold rush population boom. B.C. did have midwives, noted as late as the 1930s, but they were concentrated in the ethnic, particularly in the Japanese, populations.[9] The development of a militant nursing profession in B.C. after World War I also helped to minimize the impact of midwifery in that province.

Although midwifery was either illegal, or licensed and controlled by the medical profession in most provinces by the 1940s, it continued to exist to varying degrees in different areas. The distribution of midwives, predictably, reflected the distribution of doctors and the patterns of urbanization and industrialization across the country.

Hospital versus Home

During the 1890s the first systemized efforts were made to improve conditions at the lying-in hospitals in Ontario and Quebec. To be effective teaching centres, these institutions had to attract a higher volume and a better class of obstetrical patients. The nursing profession was by now on hand to effect the clean-up. So the push toward hospital birth that would edge the community midwife out began. She was not welcome in hospital.

Nurses, as well as doctors, resisted the presence of midwives in hospitals. The emerging nursing profession at the turn of the century had made an uneasy — and unequal — alliance with the medical profession in order to survive. Economically, the single, ill-paid, and often unemployed nurse could not afford another class of worker in the hospital.[10]

In 1919, when the first public health department was instituted, an army of public health nurses was dispatched across the nation to promote hospital maternity care. With baby fairs and baby trains they prescribed maternity and childcare: the medical way. The public health nurses were even known to provide ''incentives'' for poor mothers to go into hospitals; they gave out free layettes.

When doctors took to automobiles after World War I, the sphere of their influence enlarged. But as one New Brunswick physician is quoted in the Dominion Council of Health files:

> The automobile has practically obliterated the small village doctor. He and his representatives have migrated to the larger villages and smaller towns. Why? Because of the automobile he is now able to cover a circle or district with a diameter of between 30 and 40 miles as readily as before he covered a district of 10 miles, and still continues to charge by mileage; hence the increased proportion of non-medical attendance at midwifery cases.

The motorized physician gave midwifery a brief boost, until he began to urge his patients into hospital. His argument was focussed on modern facilities and safety. Clearly there was also the issue of physician convenience and income. Yet people followed their doctors' urgings into hospitals. It was, after all, the 1920s. And in the 1920s what was modern was best.

Medicine in the 1920s and 1930s did not offer a safer birth than the midwives. Mason surmises that a doctor's training involved observing an average of four births only.

At the 11th Annual Meeting of the Dominion Council of Health in 1924, a Dr. Seymour of Saskatchewan was firmly rebuked for having compiled maternal mortality statistics for his province. He admitted that:

> The results were not all favourable. They were such that I did not think it would have been well to give them to the public. . .a very large number of women were confined without either nurse or medical man, and the mortality among those was very much lower than those who had professional attendants. [11]

Quoting the Dean of Medicine of John Hopkins University, Dr. Seymour attributed the bad statistics to medical men not knowing their obstetrics.

The main causes of maternal mortality at the time were infection, toxemia, hemorrhage and "accidents of pregnancy." [12] The doctors did not yet uniformly apply aseptic precautions, and they did not guess the cause of toxemia. Many hemorrhages may well have been caused by aggressive third stage management; inexperienced practitioners tugging on umbilical cords to hurry placentas along. The category "accidents of pregnancy" reflected consequences of miscarriages and abortions. The midwives were not innocent of errors, but their tendency toward nonintervention was safer under the circumstances.

> The great increase in radical or operative obstetrics after 1915 appeared to be a primary cause of rising puerperal mortality, counterbalancing lives saved as the result of the introduction of asepsis and improved prenatal care. [13]

Because increased hospitalization of birth during this century was accompanied by a decrease in mortalities, medical historians frequently infer a causal relationship between the two trends. Recent analysis has disproven the causal link. [14] The decrease in maternal mortality is actually attributed to improved sanitation, nutrition, prenatal care, etc. In fact, the initial move to hospital birthing was accompanied by appalling maternal mortality statistics.

During the 1930s, public concern about maternal mortality provoked studies in New York, Aberdeen and Ontario.[15] Although the Ontario study did not separate midwife- and doctor-births as did the studies in the United States and Britain, it did make it abundantly clear why so many women still preferred their "ignorant midwives." Not only had medicine achieved no significant reduction in maternal mortality in Ontario in 25 years, but hospital births resulted in a maternal mortality rate of 5.3 per thousand, while home births had only 2.3 per thousand. Most embarrassing was the finding that rural women, who had more midwives and home births, were better off than their city sisters, who had all the "advantages" of hospital and medical care.[16]

The evidence was so damning, that had it ever reached public consciousness, it might have reversed the trend toward hospitalization. But such facts rarely got past the pages of the medical journals. More and more women chose hospital birth, to some extent encouraged by the economic constraints of the depression. Mason points out a newspaper article in 1932 criticizing women for taking up hospital beds in order to enjoy the free room and board.

The introduction of blood transfusion techniques and the use of antibiotics in the 1930s finally gave the doctors in hospital some real safety advantages. These advances offered cures for hospital-caused infections and doctor-caused hemorrhages, while obstetrical training and hospital standards gradually improved.

The Dominion Bureau of Statistics records that everywhere but Quebec, the N.W.T. and the Atlantic Provinces, hospitalization for birth topped 50% by the end of the 1930s. The Maritimes reached this half-way mark during the '40s, and Quebec, with its deep tradition of home birth and its medically licensed midwives, resisted the turning point until 1950. Newfoundland and the Northwest Territories followed along in the '60s.[17]

The Demise of Community Midwifery

Midwives disappeared first from urban Ontario around the turn of the century. In British Columbia and the Yukon, there never were very many. The last significant generation of Prairie midwives probably apprenticed during the Depression decade. An elderly Quebecoise midwife recalls that in 1942, her license was simply not renewed.[18]

In the Maritimes midwives worked for a time in cooperation with home birth doctors, until the road system improved and birth moved into hospitals. Only in Newfoundland, late entrant into Confederation in 1949, did midwifery survive as a province-wide institution as late as the 1960s.

The official death knell for community midwifery was rung in 1947, when the Canadian Medical Association resolved that physicians should take full responsibility for labour and delivery. One cannot help but note that this resolution coincided with the postwar return of military medical manpower. The doctors, like other returning veterans, needed the jobs that women had handled in their absence.

The 1948 issue of the government publication "Canadian Mother and Child," in its regular section for midwives, estimated that only 1,600 mothers would give birth without medical or nursing assistance that year. By 1953, the midwifery section of the publication was deleted altogether.

From then on, even in those isolated regions where no medical care was readily available, midwifery was officially discouraged and down-played. "There is no better index of the political power of the medical profession," one journalist points out, "than the fact that it put mid-wives out of business, even where there was no doctor to provide service.[19]

Surviving Elements

Although the tradition of community midwifery was broken, and their skills largely buried, some midwives did continue to practise through the 1950s and '60s.

Doctor-births in Newfoundland remained exclusive to the cities and company towns, because doctors could not cover most of the 1,500 tiny fishing villages around the island. These outports were too isolated to permit winter travel to the few cottage hospitals that existed. Midwives performed all the duties of local healers. In a town as large as Stephenville during the 1950s, Newfoundland sociologist Cecilia Benoit grew up with a practising midwife in her neighbourhood.

Not unlike Catherine Guertain of Montreal in 1713, Benoit's local midwife was a symbol of community democracy: "She had to show her knowledge of the women and the culture. She had to demonstrate her wisdom and her willingness. The people had to believe in her or she wouldn't be called upon."

In the 1960s, Premier Smallwood's controversial resettlement pro-gramme concentrated the Newfoundland population into a few hundred towns and a comprehensive medical health system was finally estab-lished. The midwives, no longer needed to reach where the authoritative arm of medicine would not stretch, were rapidly edged out.[20]

Within the tightly knit ethnic communities of our major cities, foreign-trained midwives continued to do home births among their own people into the 1950s and '60s, usually alongside a doctor from the old country.

Today, one still hears of an elderly Russian midwife practising in Northern Ontario, of a Hutterite midwife in Southern Alberta. But these are isolated cases.

The Inuit and Indian tribes of the North were the last cultures to retain midwifery. Protected by cold, isolation, and their distinctive lifestyles, they held on to the midwifery tradition. The unofficial communication link known as "moccasin telegraph" still whispers about native midwives active in the 1980s.

But since the Medical Services Branch of Health and Welfare Canada began to send medical personnel into Canada's far-flung Northern communities, the native midwife's activities have been largely curtailed. Medical Services itself became the final bastion of midwifery in Canada, but nurse-midwifery, rather than community-midwifery. Until 1970, Medical Services hired foreign-trained midwives to serve in its isolated nursing stations.[21] Although these nurses were never formally acknowledged as midwives, their birth work was well enough known to create the lasting public misimpression that midwifery is somehow legal above the Arctic Circle. This is not the case.

As a result of a Medical Services Branch policy "to provide services in remote areas comparable to those the rest of the population receives,"[22] midwifery is losing its last stronghold in the North. In one recent year, 1,500 women were flown out of their communities, often weeks ahead of their due dates, in order to deliver their babies under doctor supervision in Southern hospitals. Fewer and fewer of the Medical Services nurses feel confident about handling deliveries on their own.

By 1984, Medical Services had 95 nursing stations with no physician on site, and 104 nurse employees with full (foreign) midwifery credentials. Yet in 1980 they reported that only 86 of 7,500 births under the Service occurred in nursing stations. A further 141 births occurred at other locations. Perhaps nurses conducted deliveries in Native and Inuit homes, or en route to the stations? Perhaps these births were seen by native midwives or by no one at all?

For the majority of Canadians, the most persistent reminder of midwifery during its decades of dormancy has been the presence of foreign, mostly British, nurse-midwives on our obstetrical wards. Although their midwifery training is not officially acknowledged, and they are not permitted to deliver babies or to provide continuous care, they do lead the obstetrical nursing teams in many of our major hospitals.

Their role in training other obstetrical nurses is significant enough to cause concern among health care observers. When the post-World War

II immigrant wave of nurse-midwives retires, will our hospitals suffer a dangerous expertise gap?[23]

As well as thousands of these nurse-midwives, Canada has a significant population of foreign-trained midwives who are not nurses, and who therefore cannot even work in obstetrics. Together, these groups constitute a massive wasted workforce. While Canadian women militate for the kind of care these midwives might provide, the midwives stand by with their hands tied, watching their skills rust.

Revival/Rebirth

Into this climate of nurse-midwife or no midwife came the "new midwife" of the 1970s. She owes her existence to radical changes of public attitude about birth since the 1960s, and to the lack of a radical response from the hospital-medical system.

The movements and revolutions of social change that swept across North America after 1960 created a new climate of ideas conducive to midwifery. At first among the counterculture, and increasingly in the middle-class mainstream, these ideas took hold and altered parents' expectations about birth and family life.

Since the 1950s, parent consciousness and birth activism had been on the rise in North America. In the face of the dominant "knock 'em out, drag 'em out" norm of medical deliveries, the British Doctor Grantly Dick-Read's *Childbirth Without Fear*, and then the Lamaze method of natural childbirth, won increasing popularity. Parents organized to teach and learn about birth, but only the rarest kooks sidestepped the hospital system.

The West Coast back-to-the-land movement of the 1960s promoted a self-sufficient daring that allowed a few committed idealists to take birth into their own hands. Their premium on independence and their abhorrence of institutional power structures suggested home birth even when there was no doctor available. They began to go it alone. And the results were not disastrous.

This was a well-fed, hard working population, in good shape for normal birth. Most were dedicated to natural and holistic philosophies of well-being. They avoided the drugs and interventions of modern medicine in favour of a preventative approach to health. Hospital birth clashed with their lifestyle. Midwifery, they soon discovered, was a smooth fit.

Meanwhile, Eastern spiritual concepts were seeping into North American thought, bringing a new reverence for birth, life and death, and an understanding of the interaction of body, mind and spirit.

Popular psychology influenced the birth picture with the ambitions of the human potential movement and the revelations of primal therapy. Psycho-social factors that had not previously been connected with childbirth became real concerns for some parents. Even before Dr. Frederic Leboyer's *Birth Without Violence* was published in 1975, the vanguard of the midwifery movement was catering to infant sensitivities, and seeking to avoid birth trauma to mothers and babies.

At the same time, the women's movement nurtured women's pride in their bodies, and reintroduced them to their rights. Without this major sociological shift, the female midwives would never have had the support they needed to operate at odds with the powerful male medical profession.

The sexual revolution had empowered women to make their own reproductive choices for the first time. Birth style became one of those choices. Widely available birth control in the 1970s resulted in a generation of planned parents who were older, better educated, and more ambitious birthers than ever before. The information explosion gave them paperback access to research and opinions not previously available to the lay public. More parents took it upon themselves to become experts. They began to question the social and psychological shortcomings of medical birth, and then its very safety.

The halo of the medical profession was tarnishing by the 1970s. Not only were people talking about the limits to science, they were discovering that much of medical birthing routine was not even based on scientific findings.

At first, most of these new patterns of thought belonged to the outlaws and the intellectuals. The overwhelming majority of Canadian parents never questioned the only birth style they had ever known. It would take the consumer movement of the 1970s to raise the expectations of a critical minority. But once the middle classes began to assess options, demand service, and seek personal satisfaction from caregivers, there was room at least to entertain the midwifery option.

Midwifery was an alternative that responded to individual parents' beliefs. The medical maternity care delivery system, so long a monopoly comfortably supported by socialized medicine, was not ready to be responsive.

Midwifery got its foothold in most communities because hospital policies clashed with parents' wishes. Although some big city hospitals offered a narrow range of parental choices in the 1970s, most Canadians had access to only one hospital, with rules that lagged behind their birth ambitions. A Nova Scotia midwife-to-be described the restraints on birth at the only maternity hospital in her region in 1972: 1) Fathers could not attend deliveries, only labours. 2) Episiotomies were performed routinely. 3) Mothers were only allowed to be with their babies on a four-hour feeding schedule. She chose a home birth instead, flying in her midwife all the way from Vancouver.

Parents questioned unconscious cesarean sections, routine anaesthesia and analgesia, lack of support for breastfeeding. They opposed separation of newborn and parents, the insult of the obstetrical stirrups, and the humiliation and loneliness of unsupported, depersonalized hospital birth. All these "customs" contributed to the attractiveness of home birth and midwifery care. For those who needed or chose hospitalization, the idea of taking a midwife along as a protectress became popular in the latter 1970s.

The home birth choice necessitated midwives in some communities, because there were no doctors willing to attend. In other places, where a few doctors did do home confinements, midwives acted as labour sitters at first, working under the doctors' supervision. As they became more experienced, they caught babies. Sometimes the doctor was late. They took on increased responsibility. Eventually some parents, preferring a non-medical approach and a woman attendant, chose a midwife instead of a doctor.

Pioneers of the New Midwifery

> All changes come from the consumer. We weren't soliciting and creating a need. The population was already there, unattended. We were offering a service to people who otherwise wouldn't have their needs met.
>
> — Cheryl Anderson,
> Lay Midwife, M.D.

The Vancouver Free Childbirth Education Centre, spawning ground for the new midwifery in Canada, opened in 1971. Funded by the Federal government's Local Initiatives Program, it was operated by a collective of twelve, including Cheryl Anderson, lay midwife-to-be and later physician. Its mandate was to provide free prenatal education to transient West Coast youth. This was the first organized attempt to meet the needs of a growing population who opted out of the medical care system and chose to give birth at home and often unattended.

Anderson had spent two summers on a medical bus, providing prenatal care information in rural British Columbia. She wanted to learn more about prenatal education, and headed for Santa Cruz, California, where she heard people were questioning hospital-mode deliveries. Under the wing of midwife Raven Lang, Cheryl found herself learning midwifery skills. The following year, when she helped open the Vancouver Birth Centre, Anderson recruited Raven to join the staff.

Committed home birthers from all over the province came to the Centre. Inevitably, those seeking prenatal care and information began inviting Cheryl and Raven to births. After considerable discussion the Birth Centre collective agreed that it was important for the midwives to share their skills by attending births, even if that meant jeopardizing the Centre's funding. So Cheryl and Raven went to about ten births a month, sometimes along with one of a handful of home birth doctors.

The Free Childbirth Education Centre received surprising support from the medical community. The midwives visited hospitals to tell about their work, and doctors visited them to observe and consult. One obstetrician taught Raven and Cheryl about managing birth complications, and then donated all his old obstetrical texts to the Centre.

Midwife-apprentices soon began to emerge from the population of new mothers. As well as prenatal care and education, daycare and post-partum counselling, activities at the Centre in 1972 included workshops, conferences and midwifery classes. At the beginning, a woman's apprenticeship might have included attendance at ten births. Within a few years, the requisite number rose to fifty.

In February 1973, the Centre began keeping birth statistics. These are perhaps the first formal tallying of lay midwifery outcomes in North America. In one year the various midwives attended 86 home and hospital births. The only mortality was a tiny twin boy, born in hospital. The most common notations beside the home births are the words "no problem" or simply "tear."[24]

After a year at the Centre, Raven Lang had moved to Vancouver Island, nurturing a group of would-be midwives studying there. In 1974 Anderson chose to practise midwifery for her personal circles, which stretched to Quebec and Saskatchewan. The Birth Centre underwent several moves, dormancies and reincarnations during the 1970s. It continued to "graduate" new midwives, who took their expertise back out across the province.

British Columbia undoubtedly had the greatest number of active midwives during the 1970s, and the Kootenay District around Nelson, B.C. became the home birth boom centre of Canada. One study confirms that home births in that region, attended mostly by midwives, accounted for as much as eight percent of the birthing population.[25]

But the West was not the only place in Canada where midwifery was reviving. As early as 1973, the Nova Scotia Association for Prepared Childbirth harboured a midwife attending births along with a home birth doctor. A Nova Scotia home birth study group was frightened out of existence in 1975, when the Provincial Medical Board began to enquire about "non-hospital obstetrical activities."[26] (The study group format, in which a group of interested home birth mothers met regularly to share information and practise midwifery skills, launched Canadian midwives in many communties.)

Cheryl Anderson found herself in Montreal in 1974, for the usual reason: "There's always a birth that takes me places." She attended four births while working with a women's self-health group, L'Auto Santé. There were no practising midwives in Quebec yet, although some of her colleagues were attending home births as supporters.

Visiting her home province of Saskatchewan next, Anderson found a few committed progressive physicians working with some women who were becoming midwives. Saskatchewan was to be a slow-growing, but persistent pocket of midwifery activity right into the '80s.

By 1975, midwives were quietly acquiring skills in communities as diverse as Montague, Prince Edward Island, Ottawa and Calgary. Also of course, in the rural cooperatives of Ontario and Quebec.

The restrictive hospital policies in smaller centres fueled radical birth choices. Sympathetic doctors backed up the midwives for hospital care. Home birth doctors found diligent midwife "labour sitters" indispensable to their practices.

According to the minutes of a 1974 meeting of the Ontario Nurse-Midwives Association, there were some granny midwives operating at that time out of a health clinic on Dupont St. in Toronto. But most of the rapidly increasing demand for home birth in Toronto during the seventies was handled by a distinguished general practitioner, Dr. John Mc-Coulagh, and a few other physicians. Not until 1978 did the Toronto community of new midwives begin to take form.

At a public meeting of the Home Birth Task Force that year, a massage therapist stood up and enquired about how she could become a midwife. After the meeting a handful of women with similar aspirations gathered. They eventually formed a midwifery study group.

A subsequent visit by Texas lay midwife Shari Daniels was just the catalyst the would-be Toronto midwives needed. Task Force organizer Mary Sharpe recalls: "That was an important time. Shari talked to us as if we were, or could be, midwives. That got a lot of us fantasizing."

Within a year Sharpe was off to El Paso to Daniels' Maternity Center. Midwifery training there was a six month trial-by-fire, assisting poor, high risk Mexican mothers. In spite of Mary's warnings about the high stress, high risk orientation, two other aspiring Ontario midwives followed her to El Paso. Just as the Santa Cruz midwives influenced the development of the British Columbia midwives, so Daniels' school influenced Ontario midwifery.

Meanwhile, several Toronto women chose to develop their birthing skills by working with the home birth doctors. In 1979, these midwives began to hold their own prenatal care clinics, independent of the physicians. But only in 1983, when the College of Physicians and Surgeons of Ontario pressured local doctors off the home birth front, did Toronto midwives routinely attend births without physicians. In the face of their increased responsibility, they paired up for each "catch."

In Edmonton, midwifery was instigated by home birth doctor Benjamin Toane, in 1978. Practice in that city was influenced by the presence of the Advanced Obstetrical Nursing programme at the University of Alberta (one of three schools in Canada providing graduates of nursing with some midwifery training). Whereas lay midwives, led by Sandra Botting, had been practising in Calgary for years, the Edmonton public assumed that midwives were nurses. Partners Sandra Pullin and Noreen Walker soon developed the highest volume home birth practice in the country, attending as many as thirteen births in one month in 1983.

Midwifery was slow to develop in Montreal, according to the Quebecoises *sages-femmes* who began practising in 1979. Their language cut them off from the literature of the birth and midwifery movements in North America. Having only moved away from home birth within living memory, the public also tended to view it as "going back to the oil lamp." The back-to-nature ethos had not caught on in Quebec, as it had in Ontario and British Columbia. Nevertheless, in Quebec, as elsewhere, by 1984, demand for midwifery services far exceeded supply.

Also around 1979, several midwives, including two Mennonite nurses, became active in Southwestern Ontario. Midwifery re-appeared in Nova Scotia. In New Brunswick, a nursing instructor quietly attended a few friends at home. Ironically, in this one province without restrictive midwifery legislation, she appears to be the sole practitioner.

Not until 1980 did three Manitoba midwives surface. One of them regularly travels 250 kilometers from Brandon to Steinbach attending births. Her territory includes an Ojibway reservation, where she has attended births along with an elderly native midwife.

If there are any midwives in the Yukon or Northwest Territories — outside of the nursing stations and native communities — they have yet to reveal themselves to their southern sisters. And in spite of the fact that the turn-of-the-century Newfoundland Midwifery Act still stands, midwives have yet to make a comeback in that island province. Perhaps because Newfoundlanders received full medical services so recently, they are as yet reluctant to criticize their health care system.

The ranks of the practising midwives across Canada are still very small, largely due to their legal non-status. In 1984, just over one hundred midwives are actively catching babies in service to Canadian parents. But their impact has been disproportionate. The midwifery movement, amplified by the mainstream media, has projected to the public an alternative model of maternity care. The presence of even a few competitive caregivers challenges the complacency of the hospital-medical monopoly. Midwifery has influenced the medical system by arming parents with a new vision of birth to aspire to. Because of the midwives, parents dare to ask more of their doctors.

And though the practising midwives are few, their national support network has swelled to the thousands and the new midwives will not likely suffer the fate of the granny midwives. As well as community popularity, today's midwives enjoy unified strength and political savvy. The parents of the 1980s will ensure that this renaissance of midwifery endures.

Notes

1. Maude Abbott, M.D., *A History of Medicine in the Province of Quebec.*
2. C.L. Biggs, "The Case of the Missing Midwives," in *Ontario History,* March 1983.
3. Cited in C.L. Biggs, Op Cit, "Act to Regulate the Qualifications of Practitioner of Medicine and Surgery in Upper Canada," Chapter 32.
4. W.B. Howell, *F.J. Shepherd — Surgeon: His Life and His Times.*
5. Cited in C.L. Biggs, Op Cit, Letter, *Canada Lancet.*
6. Cited in C.L. Biggs, Op Cit, Harrison, M.D, "Operative Midwifery," *Ontario Medical Journal,* Vol. 1, 1982, p. 154.
7. J. Oppenheimer, "Childbirth in Ontario: The Transition From Home to Hospital in the Early Twentieth Century," *Ontario History,* March 1983, p. 40-44.
8. Cited in C.L. Biggs, Op Cit, "Report on the 11th Annual Meeting, Ottawa, December 15-17, 1924." *Dominion Council of Health Files,* Series 5, Box 1. p. 23.
9. "Annual Report of the Canadian Nurses Association," *National Council of Women Yearbook,* 1932.
10. G.M. Weir, *Survey of Nursing Education in Canada.*
11. Cited in C.L. Biggs, Op Cit, *Dominion Council of Health Files,* p. 22
12. Ibid, pp. 27-28.
13. Joyce Antler and D.M. Fox. "The Movement Toward a Safe Maternity Care," *Bulletin of the History of Medicine,* 1976, pp. 569-595.
14. Neil Devitt, "The Transition From Home to Hospital Birth in the U.S. 1930-1960," *Birth and the Family Journal,* Summer 1977, pp. 45-58.
    Marjorie Tew, "The Case Against Hospital Deliveries," in *The Place of Birth,* Oxford Medical Publications, 1978.
15. "Maternal Mortality in New York City: A Study of all Puerperal Deaths 1930-1932," New York Academy of Medicine, 1933.
16. J. Oppenheimer. Op Cit, "Childbirth in Ontario," p. 54.
17. "Number and Percentage of Births Occurring in Hospital 1921-1973," *Dominion Bureau of Statistics.*
18. Aurore Begin. Interviewed in "Depuis Que le Monde et Monde," (Film) Produced by Naissance Renaissance Montreal, 1981.
19. David Cayley, "The Medicalization of Childbirth," *Morningside,* CBC Radio, Fall 1981.
20. Cecilia Benoit, Unpublished Doctoral Research, Personal Communication, 1984.

21. Maria NcNaughton, Nursing Advisor, Medical Services Branch, Health and Welfare Canada, Personal Communication 1984.
22. D.A. Sheddon, M.D, Medical Services Branch, Personal Communication, 1984.
23. Elizabeth Hyndman-Erb, "The Practising Nurse-Midwife in British Columbia," *Midwifery is a Labour of Love,* Maternal Health Society, Vancouver, 1981, p. 36.
24. Cheryl Anderson et al, "Birth Statistics Feb. 1973 - Feb. 1974, Vancouver Free Childbirth Education Centre," Unpublished.
25. "Home Birth Information and Data Gathering Survey," Nelson, B.C., Health and Welfare Canada Project 1216-9-144.
26. M.R. MacDonald, M.D, Corresponding for Provincial Medical Board of Nova Scotia, July 8, 1975.

Bonnie Johnson

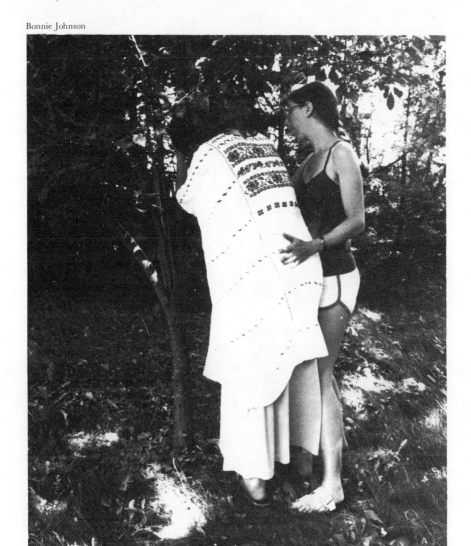

Midwife Bobbi supports Henni while labouring outdoors.

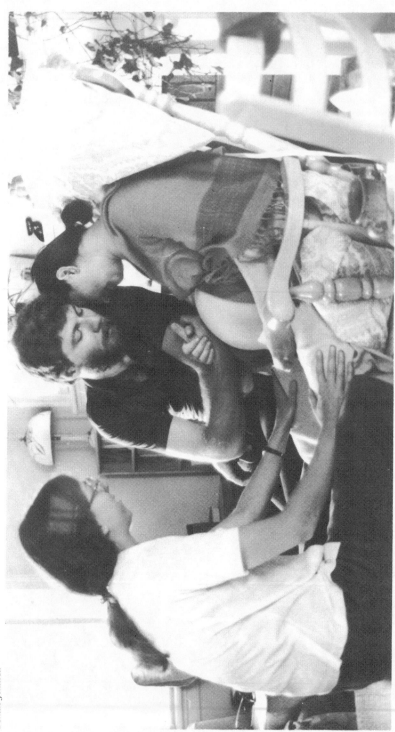

Bonnie Johnson

Bobbi and husband Scott support Henni.

Chapter Three
Vocation of Vigilance

Why be a Midwife?

I am a midwife because I was too lazy to stuff myself into molds that fit
less well. Midwifery and me. The same thing really.

— Theo Dawson

An informal survey of a dozen practising midwives reveals a
curious array of past lives: one actress, three nurses, two journa-
lists, a teacher, an occupational therapist, a weaver, an X-ray
technician, a massage therapist, and a bookkeeper. Clearly there is no
prescribed career path into this profession. All that the midwives have in
common is motherhood. The only prerequisites are life experience,
quick intelligence, a giving personality, and a passion for birth.

The discovery of midwifery is like a homecoming for some women. "I
knew in my fingertips as soon as I started feeling bellies: This was my
work," declares Cheryl Anderson, lay midwife and doctor. Like so
many of her sisters, Cheryl harkens back to her grandmother, who was
once a community midwife.

Midwifery is typically a second career, a discovery of "right liveli-
hood" that comes after post-secondary education, some other occupation, and usually parenthood. Few women take it up before the age of 25.

Rarely is it seen as an adequate source of economic support, or merely
an occupation. In the Canadian non-institutional context, midwifery is
both a calling and a lifestyle. It is an earned position in the birthing community, accredited by parents rather than by a piece of paper. The experience of birth work "pays for itself" in the estimation of some midwives.

Birth has been my teacher. It has taught me about many other
aspects of life. Medicine, healing, technology, spirituality, politics.
To be doing home births is my contribution to the world. It is my
political action. It is my spiritual discipline as well.

— Colleen Crosbie

Other midwives echo the sentiment that birth work is their personal
religion. "It is a lifestyle that requires both action and introspection,"
muses Montreal midwife Jennifer Stonier. Their dedication — or
perhaps obsession — with birthing provokes statements like this one
from Edmonton midwife Sandy Pullin: "I'll practise midwifery forever.
'Til death or jail!"

The provocations to learn midwifery are particular to individuals, but there are a few recurring themes among midwives' professional histories. The most obvious one is the enduring impact of a very good, or very bad, birth experience. Calgary X-ray technician turned-midwife Sandra Botting had both. When her first child was born the doctor's clumsy use of forceps and overenthusiastic episiotomy left her with fist-sized bruises and a torn bowel. "I couldn't sneeze, I couldn't laugh," she recalls. "I wondered if I'd ever feel anything but pain."

In hospital for her second child, she was just reaching full dilation when the doctor invited her husband to join him for lunch. Her son was born without them, and disappeared for twelve hours after. Sandra was left puzzling: "I *think* I just had a baby!?"

After her remarriage to Ron Botting, Sandra got pregnant again, and was having nightmares about hospitals. It was Ron who suggested a home birth. Sandra thought he was crazy. Until they began to read and research together. She gained confidence as they studied obstetrical texts and organized a birth support team. There were no home birth doctors in Calgary then.

Ron, a computer designer, drew flip charts for each stage of labour. Sandra called out instructions between contractions. Daughter Leda was born after an uncomplicated three-hour labour. Their fourth child, also born at home with Ron in attendance, arrived after only ten "toe curling" contractions.

Sandra participated in a home birth study group, but did not begin attending until a woman doctor started doing home births in Calgary. For several years Sandra and Dr. Underwood enjoyed an informal partnership and mutual apprenticeship. When the doctor left town, Sandra continued her birth work with apprentices.

Some women moved gradually from prenatal teaching or women's self-health groups into the midwifery field, responding to the needs of those around them. For Vancouver nurse and midwife Gale Gray, teaching prenatal classes to hospital birth couples became very frustrating: "I was telling people about how they could have their babies, then throwing them off the cliff with only a 'good luck.'" She began to feel she had to go along.

Other women were dragged into the work by accident or fate. Graduate journalist Betty Anne Putt got her "calling" in Guatemala after the earthquake in 1972. She was there to make a film, but distraught villagers kept dragging her off to premature labours precipitated by the quake. They assumed that an educated *Nordamericana* would be able to help. After a few such incidents Putt sought midwifery skills and training.

Ava Vosu was provoked to learn midwifery by a personal tragedy. Living in a small Northern Ontario town and dedicated to a natural birth for her first child, Ava could not find a supportive doctor or hospital within 200 miles. She finally had to settle for a home birth in Toronto, with a midwife who admitted that she had only limited experience. Encountering the new germs of the Kensington Market district only a few days before the birth, Ava ran a fever. An apparently healthy boy was born without mishap, but three days later, he died of an infection. Ava got a clear message: "If he died for anything, it was for me to learn midwifery and provide the skilled alternatives I couldn't find. Within three weeks I was in Texas, at Shari Daniels' Midwifery School."

Becoming a Midwife

The nature of midwifery training has been almost as variable as the motivations for it. Some simply learn by doing, others go abroad to earn foreign credentials. Apprenticeships to doctors or midwives, self-study and correspondence courses, conferences and workshops all fill some of the skills gaps.

Because there is no official training which earns one the title of midwife in Canada, most of our midwives exhibit that healthy degree of professional insecurity that keeps them seeking more knowledge. They tend to take advantage of every opportunity to increase their knowledge, be it a skills exchange workshop in town or a conference across the country. "I have never met a midwife who didn't want to know more," observes one impressed health professional.

Ideally, according to Theo Dawson who has apprenticed several midwives, a woman should develop her work through several different paths of training. Dawson feels that the "combination pizza midwife" offers her clients many strengths.

Former midwife Skye Raffard of Victoria, B.C. exemplifies the early West Coast midwife's empirical or experiential training. It began with the birth of her first child at home in 1974. She had prenatal care with midwife Raven Lang, and was attended by a fellow midwife-to-be. Nineteen years old at the time, Skye was living in the country, chopping wood, hauling water and herding goats. Her 10-½-pound baby was born without incident after a 36-hour labour. Because the local hospital in Nanaimo was notorious for its backward treatment of birthing mothers, Skye was not the only local woman to choose home birth.

Others invited Skye to their births because of her experience. "You've seen it. You'll know if there's too much blood." She looks back on some of her early births as "unsafe given the circumstances," but somehow she was never presented with problems bigger than she could cope with.

Gradually, Skye learned to manage various complications, as they came up. "You'd read about shoulder distocia," in the work group, she claims, "and the next week you'd be at a birth with shoulder distocia." There were no deaths or mishaps in her practice. Skye attended over 350 births before she moved on to nursing, to help support her family.

For those like Mary Sharpe and Ava Vosu, who chose the lay midwifery training available at the El Paso Maternity Center, there was some sense of a formal education, although it led to no recognized credentials. Sharpe came to midwifery via teaching, motherhood, La Leche League and the Lamaze organization. She had already attended 50 births in Toronto with home birth doctors when she went to Shari Daniels' to get high risk experience. Her 70 births there included diabetic and epileptic mothers, twin and breech deliveries. Because much of the clientele were poor Mexican women who slipped across the border for their births, the local hospitals would only help when a woman was visibly hemorrhaging to death. "We helped all sorts of desperados," recalls Ava Vosu.

British midwife Sue Rose, who has practised in Toronto since 1982, completed the two-year "direct entry" midwifery program in England. She was not a nurse. Her training included 100 births, and four months of apprenticeship with an older midwife, who still did some at home. After working in hospital for six months, Sue became frustrated because shiftwork did not allow her to provide continuity of care. Too many women were meeting a strange midwife when they arrived in labour. Sue chose to practice independently doing home births in London.

The closest approximation to midwifery credentials that can currently be obtained in Canada are the post-graduate obstetrical nursing courses offered at the University of Alberta at Edmonton, Dalhousie University in Halifax and Memorial University, Newfoundland. These courses are designed for nurses serving in isolated stations where they may have to take responsibility for births.

The Advanced Practical Obstetrics program at the University of Alberta lasts eight months and averages 30 births. Instructor Joyce Ralyea clarifies that it is not comparable to British midwifery training, but that the course could easily be developed to be so. Sandra Pullin and Charlene MacLellan are two U. of A. graduates who practise midwifery in Edmonton and Halifax respectively.

As more of the practising midwives developed a comprehensive base of experience, apprenticeship became the increasingly popular route to training. It adapted to the needs of the community and the circumstances of the aspiring midwife. In rural districts an apprenticeship might last several years, because there are relatively few births to attend. In Vancouver or Toronto an apprentice might accumulate enough birth experience inside of one year. Kootenay midwife Abra Palumbo chose to stretch her informal apprenticeship over many years, so that it would not interfere unduly with her young family. Toronto midwife Vicki van Wagner, who had been studying midwifery academics for two years previous, dove into birthwork with a passion. She apprenticed herself to two midwives simultaneously, and attended 50 births in ten months.

Jane Cocks' apprenticeship to Theo Dawson in 1982-83 is more usual for Toronto. Over the course of a year, Jane accumulated 3,000 hours of clinical experience, including 50 births. For the first while, she followed Theo everywhere. Observing Jane's growing abilities, the senior midwife gradually assigned her tasks like postpartum visits and hospital labour coaching.

Jane took Theo's nine-week course "The Art and Practice of Midwifery" and assisted with teaching prenatal classes. She earned her certification in cardiopulminary resuscitation through the Red Cross. In addition, Theo asked her to begin a three-year "Apprentice Academics" midwifery study programme from the United States, a course which required critical reviews of 50 books on childbirth, and then moved through all the major obstetrical texts currently studied by medical students.

Jane estimates the cost of her apprenticeship year, including daycare, books, equipment, courses, gas and mileage at about $10 thousand. Her apprenticeship ended at the pre-appointed time because she had seen and helped manage all the common complications of pregnancy and childbirth. Both she and Theo were confident in her abilities. Nevertheless, Theo, or another more experienced midwife, continued to attend all Jane's births for many months.

Midwives' Workstyles

Given these diverse routes of entry, it is not surprising to discover wide variations in modes of practice. Midwives' workstyles have developed through both choice and circumstance.

Some midwives confine their work to home births, because that is where they feel most needed, and they can cope with the volume of clients. A few do only home births because a second support person is not welcome in their local hospital. Most attend both home and hospital births, following a client to her chosen venue.

A midwife offers the client planning a hospital birth the option of home labour. When contractions begin she goes to the home to assess progress, monitor medical factors, and assist in all the usual ways. Her presence allows the parents to postpone the trip to hospital until late in second stage, barring any complications. This makes for a more intimate and relaxed labour, as well as buying time for longer births. Hospital staff tend to time labour from arrival, rather than the onset of contractions, so the couple who come late may be faced with a looser medical timetable, and therefore fewer interventions.

When a planned home birth is transferred to hospital, (perhaps 10% of the time) for failure to progress or in an emergency, the midwife will stay by the woman's side (unless experience has shown her that her presence will prejudice hospital staff against the client). In progressive hospitals, a nurse hands the midwife her cap and gown. In conservative institutions, she is ignored or shown the door. Diplomacy is a key asset of the midwife in hospital. Says Victoria "labour coach" Mea Hutchison: "I don't want power plays between the midwife and the nurse to get in the way of the happy birth. I'm not there to power play. Until things change, I'll say the right words."

Midwives may work as loners and in groups, but the general consensus is that a partnership, at least, is desirable. Years ago Skye Raffard worked by herself in an island practice that drew couples to her home in planes, motorboats and by ferry. She lived only six blocks from a hospital, so emergency back-up was available, but she looks back on the stress of those years with disbelief: "After I had a partner, I'd never do it alone again. I don't know where I grew that other pair of hands. You need one pair for the mother and one pair for the baby. Either everybody's fine or they both need help."

Working in pairs allows the primary midwife a nap during a long labour. As well as four hands and two brains, it can double the number of past birth experiences to draw on if a problem arises. Generally, one midwife or the other will recognize a problem situation. Second opinions are invaluable to midwives working in the current political climate. "We can't afford to make any mistakes," Nelson midwife Ilene Bell points out.

Describing her own team work with Judi Pustil, Ilene suggests the depth of their symbiosis. "Our partnership is incredibly non-verbal. We don't talk about what we're going to do. It just gets done."

Such is the strength of a midwife partnership that the women are often referred to in their own community as a couple. "We were such a team," reminisces rural Ontario midwife Karen Ibbitson of her work with Colleen Crosbie. "I always held her back and she pulled me forward. In our community people said 'Collen and Karen,' not 'Brian and Karen!'"

Collectives have proven to be the ideal working arrangement for some midwives. The Midwives Collective of Toronto is five women who share a clinic space, equipment, books and work schedule. While maintaining a primary and back-up midwife arrangement for each client, the collective offers a fund of resources and expertise to draw on. If a midwife isn't certain whether a belly holds twins, there are several sets of knowing hands nearby to palpate and confirm her suspicion. Each client has a number of midwife personalities to choose from, and she meets many other couples at the collective's clinics.

The collective arrangement encourages midwives to develop special areas of interest and expertise, such as birth control counselling, single parent support or herbal remedies. It provides a ready forum for workshops, professional development and peer review rounds. Perhaps most vital is the collective's function as a support group for the practising midwife, and the fact that it allows each midwife some time off. Collectives can minimize the familiar phenomenon of "midwife-burnout."

The number of clients that a midwife takes on for any given month varies widely. In addition to the births, which average about 24 hours each, she continues pre- and post-partum care for all her other ongoing clients. While some rural midwives with intimate practices catch only one or two babies a month, two Edmonton midwives regularly do at least eight. The average in Toronto is four to six primary care births a month.

Attending many births keeps her skills sharp and increases her experience with the infinite variations of labour and birth. Attending very few, she can devote a great deal of quality time to develop a deep understanding of each client. Every midwife must find her own optimal balance, if community demand for midwifery services will allow her this luxury. The needs of her family also affect the size of her practice, since not even the midwives have discovered the 36-hour day.

Some Representative Techniques

> My techniques are not a bag of tricks I take with me to births. They evolve out of my relationship with the client. Working in harmony with her is like making love, like mirroring. Through unity and symbiosis I can anticipate her needs.
>
> — Theo Dawson

Nurturing is the distinguishing aspect of prenatal care offered by a midwife. She provides a safe, open environment in which a pregnant woman can grow and explore her new state. The midwife is protective, perhaps solicitous, and available for guidance. She encourages her client through diet and lifestyle changes conducive to the development of the fetus, and psychological adjustments that help a woman welcome motherhood.

Many midwives hold that in order to nurture a new life, the sensitive pregnant woman requires extra nurturing herself. Mary Sharpe asks herself what each client might need, or want, in the way of mothering during her pregnancy and birth, and tries to provide just that.

Patience is the least obvious, and most appreciated technique of midwifery care. A midwife's vigilant presence through long hours of labour can be a great comfort. Her self-restraint in not interfering with nature's process, unless she has real reason, increases the margin of safety at her births.

The soothing use of a crooning voice, gentle touch and steady eye contact are typical of a midwife's care. Through them she communicates love, relaxation and reassurance. She demonstrates that in the deepest sense she is with the woman. Her words and touches trigger her client to let go of tension and move past pain.

Few midwives adhere to any strict pattern of breathing, like the Lamaze method, any more. Most find it more useful to suggest that women breathe fully, at whatever rate serves them best. They encourage their clients to express the power of contractions with loud noises and deep notes.

Midwives do not generally endorse a heavily disciplined approach to natural childbirth. Instead, they focus on experiencing the pain — and the progress. Declaring that labour occurs more easily when women "go with the flow," Theo Dawson once again threatens to write "The Complete Book of Un-Controlled Childbirth."

Midwives do consistently provoke their clients to move around during labour, in order to keep the pace of contractions active. They are flexible about supporting the mother in whatever peculiar position feels most comfortable for actually giving birth. A hands and knees choice may mean that the midwife works on her back with a flashlight, but that's just fine.

Visualization is a tool that more of the midwives are now making use of, either before or during labour. This psychological technique involves painting a verbal picture of how labour and birth might progress. Using the power of suggestion to pattern a woman's expectations while she is in a relaxed state, visualization appears to remove many subconscious blocks to an easy birth. Its partner technique is the midwife's incisive questioning at moments when labour gets hung up for no apparent reason. Often a woman will tell some fearful secret, or reveal an old hurt that stands in the way of accepting the imminent birth. With that off her chest, she proceeds easily.

Prolonged or inactive labour is handled in a number of creative ways. Whereas in hospital a hormone drug would be administered intravenously to stir up stronger contractions, midwives try less intrusive tricks. Perhaps the couple should be left alone to feel cozy and uninhibited together? Would he try playing with her nipples to stimulate a natural hormonal pick-up? Maybe they should go for a walk? Or make love? Or just talk about their feelings? If these things don't work, there is always a homeopathic remedy to try, or an enema. Midwives with their own infants in tow occasionally use the "borrow a baby" technique to get labour moving along. An infant sucking at the breast is often enough to stimulate a slow labour into action.

Whether she uses her traditional wooden "Pinard Horn," a fetascope, or the ultrasound dop tone that echoes the fetal heartbeat around the room, a midwife is persistent about monitoring the baby's heart and mother's vital signs. She listens often, listens right through contractions, and notes how the baby responds to the increased pressure and decreased oxygen during a strong contraction. Such skills are as essential to her work as sensitivity. She can do the work of an electronic fetal heart monitor, with considerably fewer technical foul-ups.

The traditional pride of a midwife is a perineum with no episiotomy and no tear. This saves the mother weeks of discomfort, and expresses the midwife's respect for a woman's body. It is not always possible. Nor is it essential to a safe, natural birth. But an intact perineum can be a midwife's present to her client.

It is achieved through a combination of techniques unknown to most doctors. First, the parents are encouraged to massage and stretch the vaginal opening prior to the birth, a not altogether unpleasant task. During second stage, the midwife's sterile-gloved and oiled fingers prepare the way for the descending head. Hot compresses are applied as the head crowns, to increase circulation to the vulva, thus helping the tissue stretch. The midwife coaches the mother to pant, and to measure her pushes so that the head does not slip free too fast. One skilled hand supports the perineal tissue. Instead of "flying" out of the vaginal opening, the baby can thus be gently released into its mother's waiting arms. Midwives' statistics demonstrate that, contrary to medical belief, even first-time mothers can open up enough to deliver big babies, tear-free.

The list of techniques is infinite. The tools and remedies used by midwives are an array of creative responses, some pre-eminently practical, some emotionally experimental. They do not always have to make rational sense. For a midwife to adopt a practice it just has to work and, above all, to do no harm.

Midwives' Lifestyles

The midwife's personal and professional lives are more intertwined than most, with no time of day reserved for herself or her family. Clients' personal crises and unpredictably timed labours intrude on a 24-hour basis. Each woman either copes with this or retires according to the limits of her stamina and her support systems.

Many women set out to become midwives and change their minds. The romantic allure of birthwork is rapidly offset by the exhausting hours and the emotional demands. Vicki van Wagner began her apprenticeship along with five others. Within three months she was the only student left.

Burnout is a common experience for midwives who have practised a few years. In British Columbia, where they first proliferated, there are more retired than practising midwives. Three hundred births is a commonly cited burn-out point, although at least one West Coast midwife is still working after 500.

A midwife is perpetually tied to her "beeper," her answering service, and the *&!@ telephone. She rarely dares have a drink, and only those working in collectives can leave town for a weekend. Always prepared to drop everything for a woman in labour or a new mother in distress, she makes her social commitments with the proviso: "unless there's a birth." To preserve her energy and sanity, a midwife may schedule births around a month-long summer holiday. But if a lady due in late July is three weeks late, that August vacation evaporates.

A midwife's passion for birth will carry her through all that. Not necessarily so for her family. "My kids know by now that they can't depend on me to be there," regrets one midwife who is retiring for this reason. "They're wonderful about it," reflects the single parent, "but it hurts that they can't count on me."

But the flip side of the midwife-mother who deserts her child's birthday party to celebrate someone else's "birth day," can be her availability at other times. When she's not actually attending a birth, she is usually able to work at home. Some midwives arrange to be with their children more than women who hold regular jobs.

Nevertheless, most midwife-mothers occasionally find themselves searching their souls as Theo Dawson does: "Can a midwife be a mother? Can a non-mother be a midwife? Does a mother have time to be a good midwife? Does a good midwife have time to be a *real* mother? Am I a good midwife? Am I a good mother? Am I a wife?. . .''

Living with a midwife requires flexibility, respect and self-sufficiency of her spouse. Where any of these are missing, the first casualty of practice could be her marriage or relationship. Gale Gray thought twice about taking up an invitation to apprentice. Every midwife she knew at the time was divorced. Luckily her husband is supportive of her work, and willing to take over with their two children in her frequent absences.

Sandra Botting also attributes much of her satisfaction as a midwife to the "100% support" of her husband and four children. Other couples, less lucky, bravely struggle with the special challenges of a "midwifery marriage."

The midwife's minimal income will aggravate those marital difficulties if her mate cannot afford to subsidize her community service. Practising midwifery involves significant costs. A single diagnostic instrument often carries a price tag of hundreds of dollars. Supplies, books, workshops and professional dues mount up. Many midwives find that the fees they receive barely cover costs.

The economics of midwifery are complicated by the fact that a woman who can't pay is rarely refused care. Also, midwives are often reluctant to put a price tag on their work. "How do you put a financial value on a service of love?" asks midwife Ava Vosu rhetorically, before admitting that "We *have* to!"

Midwives who support their families either come to terms with hard economic realities and up their fees, or they take a part-time job to subsidize their calling. Money and midwifery remains a touchy issue for most. Fees across the country range from free to $750. "Midwifery is a perfect field," quips Skye Raffard, "but the pay is lousy."

Adding to the time constraints, financial drain, and emotional demands involved in practising midwifery, is the fear of prosecution in the event of a death. Midwives are acutely aware of the statistical probability of a stillbirth. It could happen to anyone, regardless of their care or competence. A half-dozen Canadian midwives have endured the long public agony and expense of an autopsy or court case, only to be acquitted of any negligence. In the current political climate, a stillbirth at home is a matter for legal prosecution. A stillbirth in hospital is not. One Edmonton midwife's mate tells his kids in the morning, "If your mother isn't here when you get home, she's either at a birth or in jail." She can't quite laugh when she hears him say that.

Because of the tenuous legal status of midwifery in Canada, and the realization that midwifery is not widely available to the populations who most need it, more and more Canadian midwives feel obliged to find time for political work. They edit newsletters, organize conferences, lobby politicians and do media interviews — on top of the demands of practising.

Given all the restrictions and responsibilities involved in midwifery in

Canada today, it is difficult to imagine why anyone would continue. Yet they do. Their payoff is in personal satisfaction. Midwives enjoy a rare opportunity to participate in other people's intimate lives, and sometimes change those lives. They are paid in love, respect and learning. They are supported by networks of appreciative past clients, and buoyed up by the bright faces of the children they have brought into the world.

Sometimes midwives even win recognition within the hospital. On a half a dozen occasions, across the country, doctors in delivery rooms have deferred to lay midwives, who enjoy every opportunity to catch their clients' babies, and demonstrate their skills to hospital staff. Such acknowledgement is dear to the midwives. Veteran Vancouver midwife Lee Saxell laughs that after catching a friend's twins in hospital, she was so high she didn't have to eat for a week.

But then, for a midwife, every birth is a high. The most exhausted midwife is immediately awake when the phone rings at 2 a.m. because a client is in labour. She has an insatiable appetite for that rush of life energy that accompanies birth. Midwifery is a tough habit to kick. "We're like smokers," laughs Kootenay midwife Camille Bush after ten years of it. "We're always saying: 'I really have to quit!'"

Daniel Bianchet

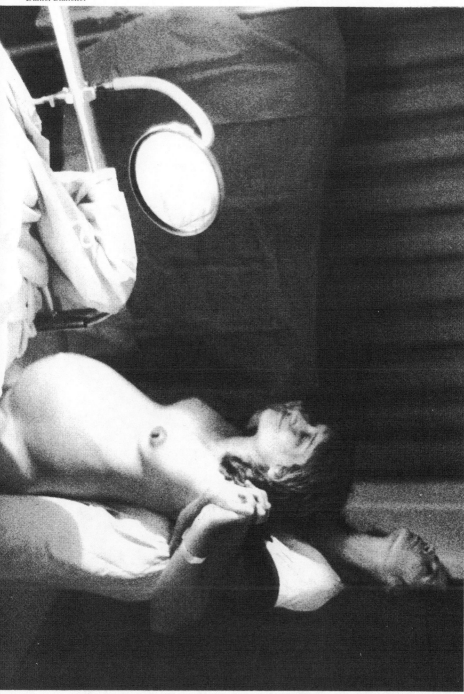

Midwife Mary Sharpe holds Beatrice in standing squat while labouring in hospital.

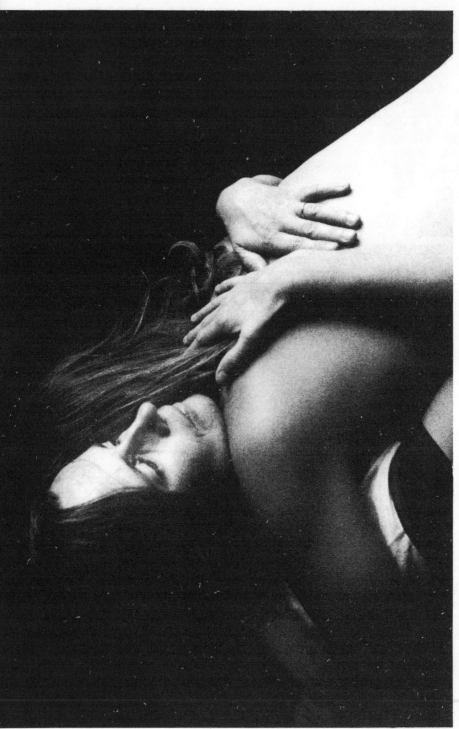

Mary comforts Beatrice during hospital labour.

Daniel Bianchet

Chapter Four
The Parents' Perspective

I used to feel like an arrow. Now I feel like a beach ball floating in hormone soup.
So I want Martin with me at doctor's appointments. I don't feel like that coming to
Mary's clinic. This is my *territory. I know you're on my side.*

— Elizabeth,
eight months pregnant

Who Hires a Midwife?

Parents who seek a midwife's services account for perhaps one or two percent of the Canadian birthing population. The great majority of pregnant couples simply proceed through standard medical prenatal care to a routine hospital birth. They are either unaware of other birthing options, can't arrange for them, or believe that alternatives like midwifery care and home birth are the foolhardy choices of a lunatic fringe.

Analysis of the current midwifery clientele denies both the designation "lunatic" and relegation to a fringe. Whereas parents who sought midwives in the early 1970s belonged to the counterculture, the current clientele is mostly mainstream. Within one decade the "hippie" ideas and birth practices spread back into the middle-class suburbs from whence the counterculturalists originally came.

A study done in California in 1974, *Birth Goes Home* by L.D. Hazell, identifies a population much like the midwifery clientele here in the latter '70s.

> The home birth set is composed of quite average people. . .approximately one tenth would be classified as "hip". . .nine tenths live in stereotypic American fashion. . . .One of the characteristics of this group is a hard to define level of self-awareness which manifests itself in an individual concern for proper nutrition and a kitchen stocked with health food, personal libraries dealing with religious topics, philosophy, positive health and humanistic psychology.

By 1984, even this vague characterization fails to catch the whole midwifery clientele. In fact, what category besides "middle class" could encompass a police officer, a fashion model, a farmer, a mathematician and a musician? Into what pigeon-hole would you file a nurse-and-dentist couple in Northern Ontario who describe themselves as "Catholic, conservative and feminist?" How "fringy" can practising lawyers and doctors and nurses be? These professions appear in significant numbers at midwifery clinics. Nurses have no illusions about what kind of attention they will get from busy obstetrical staff during their labour. Lawyers compare the midwife's advocate function in hospital with their own courtroom role. Some doctors have learned in their practices that normal birth need not be dangerous, unless medical intervention makes it so.

The midwives' clients who initially appeared as a lunatic fringe may in fact be a vanguard, those creative problem solvers who research and explore to discover a better way. One that the majority will eventually choose to follow.

Wherever midwives regularly attend hospital birthing couples, their clients include "all kinds." Some are wary consumers anxious to get the best service available. Some are single parents who might not otherwise have any personal support through labour and birth. The hospital-birthers do not have to be as radical as those choosing home birth in the current social and legal climate.

Home birth parents are perhaps more identifiable, but they too differ. Two Toronto couples, having their first babies at home with the same midwife only days and blocks apart, apparently had little else in common. The bookshelves at one house revealed the classic California home birth mindset: Gurdjieff and Wilhelm Reich and Adelle Davis. Focus on spirituality, philosophy, psychology and nutrition. The library at the other house reflected rather more materialist interests: solar heating, home renovation and gardening.

The radicalism of home birth increasingly includes religious orthodoxy. Because of the midwives' respect for the spirituality and intimacy of birth, various Christian, Jewish and Rastafarian congregations recommend their members to the midwives. One Christian group in Toronto circulates a tape of a presentation by midwife Mary Sharpe to pregnant parents.

The majority of midwives' clients are people who can afford her few hundred dollars in fees if they budget for it. But the wealthy are not immune to the need for a midwife. Vancouver and Toronto midwives report finding themselves "in the best part of town" for some home visits.

A midwife who gave private classes to an heiress and her husband at their Bayview estate was able to help the couple shed some of the aloofness of their class and culture, as well as deal with an unhappy past birth experience. When the three of them went to hospital together in labour, the midwife was pleased at how the husband was able to "really be there" for his wife. In contrast with the previous drugged birth, the mother requested only a late epidural. Her midwife was elated with the personal progress this reflected.

At the other end of the economic spectrum, some urban midwives have begun to work with the disadvantaged, who stand to benefit most dramatically from midwifery care: Single and teenaged mothers; working mothers who already have large families; those without adequate nutrition, income or support. For the most part, however, these people have no access to the information networks that lead to a midwife. Nor do they easily find the time and money for midwifery care.

Without medical insurance or institutional backing, midwifery care remains a preferred option for only those who are willing, able and equipped to search out solutions for their personal needs. The current midwifery clientele has above average education, a middle-class income, and the time and inclination for both parents to get involved in a pregnancy and birth.

Nevertheless, midwifery is gradually becoming more accessible in some parts of Canada, and as networks spread word about the midwives, the clientele no longer need to be the determined seekers that they once were. Today women hear a midwife's praises sung over the back fence, and they want one too. "There's been a mushrooming lately," observes Toronto midwife Catherine Penz. "People keep coming to me late in their pregnancy, saying they've just heard that we midwives exist. . . .All kinds of people."

Why Parents want a Midwife

Any couple who hires a midwife has some need they feel won't be met by the conventional maternity care system. Otherwise why would they pay for her services, and take the time for clinic visits? But all needs are very different. No two women reply to the "Why a midwife?" question in quite the same way:

> "I wanted her for support, continuity and camaraderie."
> — Catherine, Toronto

> "She has more skill."
> — Evelyn, Komoka, Ontario

> "She is a woman and she knows how a woman feels. She is more open to questions than a doctor. She is more available."
> — Andrée, Moncton

> "We need someone who is not too emotionally involved and who knows how the hospital works."
> — Ann, Calgary

> "I wanted humane care for a basic human event."
> — Christine, Toronto

"Home was preferable to hospital."

— Louise, Teeswater, Ontario

Midwifery care allows families their freedom, their intimacy, their sensibilities and their individuality. It can protect them in weakness, as well as developing strength. The midwifery model allows parents to creatively construct their own optimal birth scenario.

In a letter to the College of Physicians and Surgeons of Ontario in 1983, some parents described why they want midwives:

(1) She is a woman who shares our views and feelings about birth.

(2) She sees us frequently during pregnancy and spends a great deal of time with us at each visit getting to know us as individuals. This helps us to be relaxed and confident before, during and after giving birth.

(3) She stays with us during our entire labour and delivery — watching, monitoring, supporting, making suggestions and patiently waiting. This decreases the risk that any developing problem will go unnoticed.

(4) She is available 24 hours a day before and after our birth to listen, counsel, answer questions and offer support.

(5) She becomes a friend who through knowing us can help if we have emotional difficulties that interfere with the birth process or the early weeks of parenting.

(6) Several studies have shown that despite the acknowledged risk of not having immediate access to up-to-date technology, home birth with an experienced midwife is a safe alternative in childbirth.

Couples tend to cite several reasons for seeking their midwife out, and reflect differing priorities in these reasons. As well as those mentioned in the letter, parents talk about:

1) Her focus on natural birth and the safety of her non-interventive care.

2) The information and resources she shares as an equal.

3) Her understanding and involvement with the whole family.

4) Her awareness of the psychological impact of birth on the infant and parents.

The most frequently cited reason for seeking out a midwife, and perhaps also a home birth, is an unsatisfying previous birth experience. Often these are women who approached their first birth feeling confident in the conventional childbirth mode, and were shocked when things "went wrong." Catherine Penz relates the tale she hears so often at the Childbirth Education Association in Toronto: "I don't know what happened to me. I was all set. Well-educated. I did my reading. Went to Lamaze classes. . . .I like my body and I wanted a healthy baby. . .and I wound up with a cesarean! What hit me?"

The VBAC (vaginal birth after cesarean) mothers are always among a midwife's most enthusiastic clients. About one fifth of Canadian babies are now born by cesarean, and most of these mothers are faced with the "once a cesarean, always a cesarean" dictum when they get pregnant again. A home labour, carefully monitored by a midwife, often stretches past nervous hospital policy to ensure that the trial of labour has a fair chance of ending in a vaginal birth. The VBAC mother especially needs all her midwife's confidence, and freedom from the pressure of deadlines, in order to believe that her body can indeed deliver.

"You realize why you want a midwife after you've had an unnecessary cesarean," comments a Calgary mother who had that experience. But most women don't deal with their sadness and dissatisfaction about a birth immediately. When the baby is born, mother is too preoccupied with its needs to consider her own feelings, even if she is suffering postpartum depression. Perhaps a year later, when someone describes a more fulfilling birth, or a similar personal disappointment, the old pain flows back in and demands examination. "It wasn't until much later that I started to feel gyped," announces a second-time pregnant mother at a midwife's clinic. Sometimes a subsequent pregnancy triggers delayed disillusionment with a maternity care system that somehow failed the woman first time around and she considers the midwife option.

Not all motivations for seeking a midwife are deemed desirable by the caregiver. Midwives actively discourage those who come demanding a home birth simply because they are ideologically opposed to hospitals. All home birth clients are encouraged to plan for the possibility of hospital birth. Any experienced midwife appreciates medical facilities in appropriate circumstances. Several assert that it is always the couples who are "allergic to hospital" that end up needing one.

Trendiness brings some parents to the midwife's door. "It's embarrassing," admits Kootenay mother Maureen, who is now a well-informed midwifery advocate, "but I don't know why I wanted my first baby at home. I had no strong reasons. It was the culture. . .my friends." The danger with trend followers is that they are not always highly motivated to take on responsibility for their birth. Thus they, too, are encouraged to opt for hospital, with the midwife.

But a surprising number of midwives' clients do arrive at their first visit having read a dozen childbirth books, and have developed a clear cut picture of their goals and their midwife's role. They come to her precisely in order to retain control over their childbirth experience. They have weighed safety and risk and psycho-social factors and arrived at birthing decisions that best suit the balance. Their choice of a midwife is a reflection of their active concern for the quality of life that their baby will enjoy.

Finding/Choosing a Midwife

> I have spent countless hours in an absolutely fruitless search for a home birth attendant. . . .Women like me must be totally prepared to go it alone, without the benefit of adequate medical obstetrical advice, and without a trained birth attendant. In a modern urban city this is deplorable.
>
> — Shere, Windsor, Ontario

The files of midwifery organizations are filled with such anguished cries from parents who cannot find the birth support they need. Some have engaged in lengthy correspondence around their province, only to find that there are two or three practising midwives. One is pregnant herself, one has too many births to dare travel near this woman's due date. The last won't attend without a familiar doctor for back-up. Faced with a situation like this, some people actually move. A woman who uprooted her family from Calgary to Vancouver to find a midwife warns others that nine months may not be enough time to arrange for the birth support they need.

Others import a midwife. A couple living in Northern Saskatchewan chartered a bush plane to fly their midwife down from her nursing station in the Territories.

> We spent $3,000 of our own money to have the kind of birth and birthing attendant we desired. . . .We would do it again. . .to achieve such a totally positive experience.
>
> — Mary, Kinoosa, Saskatchewan

In Southern Ontario and Southern British Columbia, where practising midwives are most concentrated, one phone call to a local childbirth organization might result in a list of midwives' numbers. There is no yellow pages listing yet, but parents in areas where midwives have enough consumer support to come out of the closet are spared a frustrating search. Instead, they can concentrate their energies on the choice of the most experienced and appropriate midwife.

It is hoped that the appendices to this book: "How to Find a Midwife" and "How to Choose a Midwife" will be of direct aid to parents facing either situation.

En/Countering Disapproval

Parents who hire a midwife or choose a home birth step outside the current norms of our culture. They often unwittingly make themselves targets for righteous defenders of the status quo. Most can expect curiosity, judgement, even hostility, from well-meaning acquaintances. Sometimes the most powerful opposition comes from those they love best.

The decision to take a midwife into hospital may provoke only curious "Why?s" from friends and relatives. But it can involve challenging hospital policy to win entry for a second support person. The doctor and the nursing staff may feel threatened. People will ask if the midwife is really worth all this trouble.

Home birth parents encounter more serious disapproval. Most people still implicitly trust the medical system. They honestly believe that hospital is the only place of safety, despite the lack of data to support this position. (See Chapter Eight.) They feel obliged to try to dissuade their friends from the "rash act" of a home birth, believing the parents to be selfishly placing their own personal experience above their baby's well being.

An obstetrician's son shoulders his father's accusation that he and his wife are planning a "heinous crime," a home birth. A sensitive, pregnant young woman cries in her midwife's arms because her own mother is threatening a heart attack over the home birth plan. Couples decide not to tell anyone about their birth plans because they are tired of having to explain and defend their well-reasoned choices. Why provoke all that negative energy? An Alberta woman recounts in amusement how she overheard two ladies in the laundromat discussing "some crazy woman who was going to have a baby at home." She realized they were talking about her.

Public reaction of this kind is usually based on genuine concern, mixed with ignorance. Parents inevitably share in the midwife's constant task of public education, and one of their midwife's more valued functions is reassurance. "I'm not so strong that I can't be influenced by other people's doubts," admits Diane, who had her first child at home in 1984. Other couples in prenatal class buoyed her faltering convictions and visits with midwife Mary gave her courage. "I always left her house with a light step."

Fathers and Midwives

Throughout pregnancy, birth and early parenting a father may undergo dramatic emotional changes that society rarely acknowledges. His relationship with his partner is altering; she may be making new demands on him. The baby often means additional career and financial pressure. At the same time, he wonders if he is qualified to be a good father. Just as a woman needs nurturing from her mate, her midwife and her friends in order to adequately nurture her growing baby, so a "pregnant" father needs extra support in order to meet his family's needs.

In prenatal visits, a midwife is anxious to see both parents so that she can respond to the man's spoken or unspoken concerns, as well as the woman's. During labour and birth, some fathers need as much support as their wives do. They feel so deeply, and give so much to their wives, that they *do* go through labour. "I couldn't have done it without you!" one father gratefully acknowledged Theo Dawson's constant consideration. "Of course *he* had the baby!" laughs Theo.

In the hospital context, a midwife helps the father stand up for birthing choices. She is there to assess each situation knowledgeably, and to advise him. "What do I know?" asks one man, grateful for his midwife's part in an upcoming hospital birth. "What am I going to say when the doctor tells me we need a cesarean or the baby will be compromised. No?!!"

Most fathers have never been to a birth before their own first. They are afraid, unfamiliar with hospital behaviour codes, and easily alienated from their mates by confident professionals and sterile procedures. "Can I hold her hand?" a man wonders, as he stares at the intravenous tube attached to his wife's wrist. "Where can I stand?" he asks, looking at all the imposing technology arranged around her bed. A midwife directs him to a safe spot by his wife's side. Tells him what he might do. Insists that he belongs.

The change in hospital policy that gave fathers entry into labour and delivery rooms has been a great boon to families. But was it indeed a coincidence that the father was "let in" just when the nurse needed to be "let out" of her traditional support role? Obstetrical procedures and technology were eating up more and more of her time. The provision of comfort measures and psychological support that was once the duty of a trained professional nurse now usually falls to the father, who may not be experientially qualified. Nursing instructor Ellen Hodnett, assessing the efficacy of the midwife's role in her doctoral thesis, points to this as another reason why mothers and fathers deserve midwives.[1]

Ideally, a father is freed of responsibility for practical measures and politicking with medical professionals, in order to concentrate his energies on loving his wife. In that capacity, no one else present is more qualified.

At home births, fathers rely on their midwife's skills and safety record. In the early days of the home birth movement men asserted their right to deliver their own babies. But as competent midwives became available, most fathers were glad to delegate the more skilled functions, preferring a relaxed emotional participation in the event.

Some men do welcome the opportunity to take both emotional and practical responsibility around births.

Instead of being that one step back, you're on the spot with everyone else. Males are insulated from the stark realities of life. At a
home birth you have to really be there.

— Jim, Slocan, B.C.

Many men find it harder than their wives do to go against the norms of
medical birth, or to question a doctor's authority. They are fearful of
birth as the unknown, or programmed to operate within male professional power structures. But once they are persuaded, and enjoy a
"radical" birth experience, these male converts often become zealous
midwifery advocates. A Vancouver newspaper editor describes his
change of mind.

I was frankly laissez-faire. Wendy felt so strongly that I was basically respecting her viewpoint. . .'till we started getting into it. Then I
realized she was *right!*

— Ian

Service and Satisfaction

Having found or chosen a midwife, a family may not, as the song says,
always get what they want. But chances are they'll get what they need.

Midwives are not saints or psychics. Their clients are not universally
satisfied. Five out of 80 Toronto mothers followed by Hodnett's doctoral
study expressed some dissatisfaction with their midwifery service.
(Compared to 22 of 80 from the nursing care group) The client's feeling
of satisfaction is the midwife's best measure of her own effectiveness. For
every family there are different goals to define and standards to satisfy.

Satisfaction with midwifery care in one Vancouver study is summarized as the result of "time available for visits, continuity of care, and
availability of the trusted caregiver. . .all traditionally related to midwifery care."[2]

In the Hodnett study, mothers who had midwives rather than nurses
attending them during labour anticipated and experienced greater
control; were more pleased with professional support; were more
pleased with their own behaviour; and had significantly more intact
periniums.

These generalizations help to legitimize midwifery for the scientific
community, but the intimate recollections of mothers and fathers speak
more eloquently to other parents. Each quote highlights some aspect of a
midwife's attentions that struck the individual as special.

The biggest part is her steadfastness. She is always there, although
things may be happening in *her* life.

— Maureen

> They gave us an hour and a half every visit. We'd talk about anything and everything. We were opening up to becoming a mom and a dad.
>
> — Barbara

> When you're with a midwife during labour, she puts her face right close. She breathes every breath with you. She's inside you. Doctors cheer you on like they were at a baseball game, but they're not holding the bat with you like a midwife.
>
> — Barb

Respect for the rights of parents to their newborn, and vice versa, is an oft-mentioned quality of midwifery care. Whereas in hospital "the un-born child belongs to the obstetrician and the newborn belongs to the pediatrician," at a midwife birth it "belongs" to the parents. She under-stands the postpartum bonding period will affect their ability to relate to the child.

> I'll love her for the rest of my life. She put him on my chest so no one could see his sex and she whispered to me, so that I could announce: It's a boy!
>
> — Jane

Personal control was the key to satisfaction for one mother having her second baby. At her first traditional hospital birth she had felt others were in charge.

> I had 95% of what I wanted, but I was still at the mercy of my doctor and hospital staff. I felt that at any moment they could pull the rug out from under me. They were still in control. They only *let* me have what I wanted.
>
> — Simone

The planned home birth for her second child moved to hospital on her midwife's advice. Despite the change of plan, Simone felt more satisfied with this second, more complicated birth. Her midwife stayed and ac-tually caught the baby. She never felt she was losing control.

An Ottawa couple who are both blind planned a home birth for much the same reason as other parents. But they had additional cause to avoid hospitals. How could they walk about during labour if her seeing eye dog wasn't allowed? How would the dog take to the new baby if he wasn't around for the initial birth and bonding period? And wouldn't the hospital staff be more likely to paternatistically take over for a blind couple?

Midwife Bobbi Soderstrom helped them persuade a doctor to attend the home birth, because of their special needs. She planned extra post-partum visits while they learned to handle the baby. And because they couldn't see the illustrations in the childbirth books, she improvised demonstrations. Bobbi used dolls and a knitted uterus to help them "feel" the stages of labour. "She's really resourceful," the clients admire. "No doctor would have the time and inclination to do all that."

Midwives are able to solve many such personal difficulties. When a mother is having trouble establishing breastfeeding, an overnight visit makes a world of difference, according to those who have endured the fear and anguish of not being able to feed their hungry baby. La Leche League midwife Mary Sharpe has a host of practical tactics, and occasionally even trades babies with a new mother, to establish that the infant *can* suck, and that the mother has indeed got milk. The midwife's role of encouraging confidence and relaxation is key to dealing with this difficult situation.

Midwives' prenatal classes are sometimes a subject of special praise. Because she is not affiliated with any institution, the midwife is free to present all the childbirth choices and to recommend even the controversial childbirth books like Suzanne Arm's *Immaculate Deception* and Cohen and Estner's *Silent Knife*. She deals with pregnancy and birth as part of a sexual continuum, and of family life. As well as meeting with other prospective parents in a homey environment, the classes offer a realistic rehearsal of what labour and birth may be.

> The essence of those classes was that you do what makes you feel good. They encouraged us to be ourselves. We heard about people who sang out loud, or just stomped around. And the slides made me really feel what it was going to be like.
>
> — Diane

During labour and birth the midwives' very presence is a boon to some mothers:

> When they arrived, I felt more free and relaxed. . .much more centred. I knew there was love and caring, combined with experience and attention. My trust in their concern and help freed me to concentrate fully on my efforts.
>
> — Christine

One father, left alone in hospital with his wife because policy kept their midwife waiting outside, gratefully recalls how she helped him via telephone. "My wife says she wants a cesarean! What should I do?" he pleaded over the line. "Don't say yes or no," the midwife advised. "Just tell her how well she's doing. How far she's already come. She'll thank you later." She did. And he couldn't thank his midwife enough for that advice.

Another pearl of invaluable midwifely advice is recounted by an amused mother in Kitchener. She didn't know what to do about the sugar water hospital staff kept bringing her to feed her newborn and she didn't feel like making waves by refusing it. Her midwife replied seriously that there was only one solution: "Why you dump it into your flowers, dear, of course!"

Humour and enthusiasm are invaluable traits in a midwife, according to parents who look back and laugh at difficult moments over which their midwife carried them. But most appreciated is a midwife's special capacity for simply caring.

Some clients express appreciation in an equally warm way. Mary Sharpe received this ultimate accolade from her client's mother, stuffed into a new pair of slippers, along with two $100.00 bills: "There is so much love coming from your heart all the time, that I wonder if your feet are cold."

Notes

1. E.D. Hodnett, "The Effects of Person-Environment Interactions on Selected Childbirth Outcomes of Women Having Home and Hospital Births," Doctoral Thesis, University of Toronto, 1983.
2. B.K. Wittmann et al, "Hospital-Based Midwifery Care — Preliminary Results," Presented at the Annual Meeting of Obstetricians and Gynaecologists of Canada, Vancouver, June 1983.

Chapter Five
The Course of Caring

Wendee and Peter

Midwifery care almost always follows certain signposts; there is a schedule of prenatal visits, continuous support through labour and delivery, and postpartum counselling. But the actual course of caring is individuated by parents and midwife. Like any developing relationship, it responds to feelings and events and is never entirely predictable.

When Wendee Wood and Peter Nasmith generously offered to share their experience under the care of midwife Jane Cocks with me, we decided that their encounter with midwifery would form this chapter, regardless of what the path of care and what the birth outcome. They were the only couple I observed with such intimate consistency. I hope that through the particulars of this midwife-couple relationship, the possibilities for many others will be suggested.

Introductions by Peter

"When Wendee was born 'Why?' was the first word out of her mouth."

"I am independent to the extreme of self sufficiency."

"Jane? In one word: patience."

Wendee and Peter married young and are proud to have kept their relationship alive over thirteen years. They were both 33 years old in 1983, at the onset of their first pregnancy. Wendee is a community recreation planner; Peter a self-employed photographer.

Wendee is pre-eminently practical, curious and determined; Peter is the artistic "let it be" balance in this relationship. While his handsome bearded presence is protected by a shy reserve, Wendee's spare 5'5" frame barely contains her enquiring personality.

Both of them are outdoors enthusiasts. Skiing, hiking, even winter camping are their shared adventures. Together with their beloved Samoyed "woofs," Nanou and Saint, they inhabit a renovated house they own in Toronto's fashionable Beaches community.

When parenthood finally became part of their life plan, Wendee and Peter proceeded together with great enthusiasm and curiosity. Thus far, pregnancy has been for these opposites attracted a rare period of easy harmony in their relationship.

Jane Cocks, their chosen midwife, is 32 years old and mother of four-year-old Parrish. University-educated as a journalist, Jane was a founding member of a cooperative community near Kingston. After teaching prenatal classes there for several years, Jane, her husband Larry, and son Parrish moved to Toronto so she could apprentice with veteran midwife Theo Dawson. After an intense year involving 3,000 hours of clinical experience and some 70 home and hospital births, Jane began taking on her own clients as primary midwife in spring of 1983. Theo continues to supervise her home births.

Jane and Larry (who is the unique male apprentice midwife on the Canadian scene) teach prenatal classes together at their townhouse. They live only a few miles away from Wendee and Peter.

Why a Midwife?

> For me, the midwife came second to the idea of home birth. I knew a couple who had their second child at home. . . .I'm a renegade at heart and willing to explore the alternatives that come up. I'm *not* doing this because it's the latest fad.
>
> — Wendee Wood

Wendee knew there were midwives around because she'd read about them in a Canadian health magazine. Through a friend of a friend she got names, phone numbers and an encouraging recommendation to Jane Cocks. Although she was very committed to natural childbirth and interested in the home birth that only a midwife would safely facilitate in Toronto, it took her several months to find time to follow up on her initiative. An insensitive pronouncement by her first obstetrician, following his routine ultrasound at eight weeks, provoked her into action.

> He said I had a low-lying placenta. That meant a 50/50 chance of cesarian. He just announced it and walked out, didn't spend any time allaying my fears.

Wendee changed obstetricians, had another ultrasound, and then called Jane for an appointment. She was later to regret having made those moves in that order.

Prenatal Visit #1 — Friday, November 18. 20 weeks.

Settled on the bed amidst the teddy bears in Jane's son's room, Wendee and Peter trade questions with the midwife. This first visit is a time to talk. Wendee tells her pregnancy story to date. Peter asks about the specifics of Jane's experience. Jane describes her services and fees. Wendee opens a file and takes notes.

Jane charges $375 for complete prenatal, birth and postpartum care, whether in home or hospital. In the event of a home birth, Theo, as second midwife, charges $150. For a series of nine three-hour classes Jane and Larry charge $90. Wendee can expect to spend $10 to $30 on birthing supplies like disposable diapers and oils if she wants to labour at home.

Time also to allay concern about that low-lying placenta: At eight weeks, Jane suggests, the placenta had little room to be elsewhere. Too early to imply a problem. Wendee's second obstetrician has said the same.

Time to get used to each other: Wendee inadvertently speeds her bonding process with this midwife by bursting into tears. The wayward Samoyed Saint is lost. Jane sympathizes.

Offering them an informed consent contract to consider, Jane suggests Wendee and Peter talk alone before making a commitment to work with her. Will this relationship meet their needs?

Like most subsequent visits with Jane, whose practice is not yet full, this appointment is open-ended. It lasts ninety minutes.

Wendee and Peter come to an easy decision. Within days she calls Jane for another appointment.

"Regardless of whether I have a home or hospital birth, I want Jane as my midwife. She's willing to facilitate either way."

Prenatal Visit #2 — Friday, December 9. 23 weeks.

> It's not that I don't feel involved, but I am an outsider, a bystander.
> It's happening to Wendee's body.
> — Peter

This visit opens into Peter's feelings about pregnancy and the birthing decisions. Wendee has read a dozen books, but he avoids the literature, not wanting to colour his personal experience with other people's notions. He is uneasy about home birth, and tries to voice his very real emotional concerns logically, in the face of Wendee's reasoned enthusiasm.

Jane opens their prenatal care file, making precise notations on her chart (See page 70). Explaining the reason for each procedure, she checks Wendee's weight, blood pressure, and urine, measures the height of her uterus, and palpates the blossoming belly to determine the baby's position. Although the obstetrician said Wendee's baby was in a breech position, head up, at the last visit, Jane's diagram shows baby's head just above the pubic bone. Perhaps it has turned over?

Prenatal Care Record

NAME _Wendee Wood._

LMP _conceived July 3_ EDD _March 27 – April 7._

PPW 102.

Visit	Date	Weeks Gestation	Urine	Weight	Pulse/BP	FHR	Position	Fundus	
2	Dec 9/83	24.	No gluc. ph.6.0	116	90/55	144	⌣⊙	24	Pelvis: physical – very fit. heart lungs abdomen good abominals talked about diet re: glucose
3	Jan 13/84	28	tr gluc tr protein ph.8.0	120	90/55	160	x	30	Hmg. 7.2 (from doctor?) working on iron in diet, also needs to increase calories, baby feels wiry. Peter: 130/90
4	Feb 10/84	32	tr gluc tr protein ph.6.0	120	95/60	132	x	31	Hmg 11.0. very active baby constipated
5	Feb 24/84	34	tr gluc tr protein ph.6.5	125	95/60	144 w/ movement	x LOP	36	pubic arc 90°+ spines blunt sacral prom fine. cervix soft. 130/80.
6	Mar 2/84	35	tr gluc tr protein ph fine	126	100/65	144.	x	36.	long talk re: home/hospital
7	Mar 16/84	37	fine	127	100/60	160 w/ movement	xxx OP	37½	Hg 13.2 Wendee thinks 10 days late.
8	Mar 23/84	38			100/60	140		37	Home visit

Possible discussion: Illnesses, symptoms, doctor visits, diet, supplements, reading, exercising, rest and sleep, back-up preparations, sexual relationship, guests and other attendants, father's role, nipple preparation, etc.

After she listens to the baby's heartbeat with her fetoscope, Jane turns the earpiece over to Wendee, then to Peter. They beam at this reassurance of their baby's healthy presence.

Jane's questions about Wendee's eating and exercise habits elicit encouraging responses. She practices yoga, and eats little of the very best foods. Her problem in the pregnancy has been lack of appetite. Not even Peter's homemade bread tempts her. Recalling Wendee's history of anorexia Jane suggests natural ice cream, an extreme measure to up the calorie intake.

Paper work begins. Jane provides a sheaf of information handouts from early pregnancy classes that Wendee and Peter have missed. She asks them to fill out forms on medical history, a week-long menu record, pregnancy notes, and birth hopes.

All three of them sign Jane's contract. Then Jane and Wendee arrange to visit the obstetrician together to discuss Jane's role and the birth plan. They prepare a list of questions.

Prenatal Visit #3 — Friday, January 13th. 28 weeks.

> He said, "you don't have to have any episiotomy, if you want to end up with a baggy bum." He does routine enemas and rectal examinations and uses forceps all the time. And he made me feel like I was the villain for asking those questions!
>
> — Wendee

After a discouraging visit to obstetrician #2, Jane and Wendee drove directly to Peter's studio to relate the details. Peter is dubious about taking up the obstetrician search again. Jane's advice: "Keep looking till you get the answers you want." She recommends an obstetrician at Toronto General Hospital who respects parents' wishes and cooperates with midwives. Peter and Wendee arrange to see him together on February 20th.

After the regular physical check-up, indicating all is well, Jane takes Peter's blood pressure too. His is the higher. His weight is up too, Peter laughs. The ice cream was a great idea!

Prenatal classes begin Tuesday, January 31st for seven weeks.

Prenatal Visit #4 — Friday, February 10th. 32 weeks.

> My biggest fear about hospital birth is getting there and having to battle. What if the doctor barges in and takes over like a sergeant-major?
>
> — Wendee

Discussion about a friend's recent birth, and the kinds of people in prenatal class. Then focus on Jane's detailed analysis of Wendee's nutritional intake. The diet is excellent but she could use more iron and as much as 600 calories more. Is she eating that ice cream? Peter grins and indicates *he* is.

The physical check evolves into an emotional check-up on the contentious "home or hospital?" question. Peter tries to express his fear of losing his wife or much-wanted child. Wendee's eyes fill as he speaks. They leave the issue at a fond impasse. They will see Jane twice in February and weekly in March.

Prenatal Visit #5 — Friday, February 24th. 34 weeks.

> Feel these pointy bones?. . .That strange sensation is the ligaments. . . .Now I'm running up your sacrum to feel what the curve is like. There's lots of room there. . . .Your cervix is very mushy and pregnant. . . .Now that's your pubic arch and this back here is your tailbone. . . .You have a very nice pelvis. We're not going to worry about you.
>
> — Jane, Internal Exam

Sterile-gloved, Jane performs an internal exam, describing as she feels. Wendee, propped up on pillows, one leg resting on Jane's knee and the other on a convenient teddy bear, remains relaxed.

Jane now has a mental picture of the path this baby will follow, and she contradicts a doctor's casual comment that Wendee might not be big enough for her baby.

Peter reports in relief that the visit with obstetrician #3 was encouraging: "He was more approachable. He invited me into the examining room. And it was he who broached the questions about what we wanted." Wendee is equally pleased, but wants to know why he phrased his acceptance of their home birth option as he did. Wendee's paraphrase of obstetrician #3: "I can't condone home birth, but I will be your back-up. You decide with Jane the venue, and let me know."

Jane explains that he must protect himself from the disapproval of medical colleagues. His position on some birth issues is considered radical. She asks Wendee to request a full blood work-up at the next visit with him, and meanwhile checks her hemoglobin.

Now that they are comfortable with an obstetrician who is on 24-hour call, the hospital birth option is less threatening. And if all continues medically well for the home birth Wendee still wants, this obstetrician would be available for telephone advice to Jane, or to meet them at the hospital in case of transfer. Jane encourages them to make a decision soon. She does not feel comfortable doing a home birth without full parental solidarity, given the legal circumstances of midwifery practice.

Prenatal Visit #6 — Friday, March 6. 35 weeks.

> This whole experience is about the child. Because there isn't any child right now, we've reached an impasse.
>
> — Peter

The home-hospital question is still unresolved, but to keep the home birth option open, Theo has been invited to attend this appointment. Wendee and Peter should get to know their back-up midwife. Theo has 250 births to her credit. She arrives with her 13-month-old son Shannon, who preoccupies a delighted Peter for most of this visit.

For Theo's benefit, Wendee runs through her fears about hospital births and her tender home birth scenario, with the baby next to her's and Peter's skin. Peter admits that in spite of the evidence, he feels safer about hospital, and that he is most nervous about how he will act. Jane points out that his responsibility to stand up for Wendee's wishes will be heavier in hospital. As a non-status midwife, she cannot speak for them directly to hospital staff.

Empathizing with Peter's concerns, Theo suggests an unusual concession to midwifery policy: they can leave both home and hospital options open. Both midwives will support them labouring at home. Since their doctor is flexible, they can simply stay home and have Jane catch the baby if that feels right at the time.

Tension dissolves into laughter at the excuse of young Shannon's antics. Theo palpates Wendee's belly to "get to know" this baby. Everyone feels the due date, April 6, rapidly approaching.

Prenatal Visit #7 — Friday, March 16th. 37 weeks.

> I'm not prepared! You'll have to show me how to change a diaper.
>
> — Wendee

Parenthood is ever more imminent and Wendee's course of reading has moved into the baby literature. She discusses her strategy for winning a six-month leave of absence from work to breastfeed this baby. It appears she may have a battle to hold her job.

She and Peter are now working every evening at gently stretching her vaginal opening, as Jane suggested in class. Wendee is determined to have neither an episiotomy nor a tear. Peter jokes about having over-worked fingers.

Wendee has become involved with the progress of other mothers-to-be in prenatal classes, comparing her own experience. She enjoyed seeing slides of many different home and hospital births, and a video of Theo delivering Shannon. She no longer feels afraid of the pain of childbirth. Her concern is focussed on creating a birthing situation where *she* feels in control.

Once again the physical check-up reveals no worry signs. Wendee hasn't gained much weight but baby has nevertheless grown to a good size, Jane estimates while palpating. And baby is in the normal head down position, allowing for a home birth.

Aside from constipation, alleviated by oranges and club soda, and frequent night voyages to the bathroom, Wendee has no complaints.

Peter, by now an expert with the fetoscope, tunes in to his baby's heart beat. He has cancelled a camping trip this weekend, not wanting to be away from Wendee so close to her due date.

Home Visit — Friday, March 23rd. 38 weeks.

> The main thing is to listen to your body. When you get crampy and achy feelings, stop right then! Don't wait till the end of the day to stop. Keep working, but if you have to work, get a good massage. You have to decide what feels nice for you.
>
> — Jane

Peter is concerned that Wendee is still working too hard, not getting any extra rest. She protests that this is her last week of evenings, but she is going to work right up to her due date on April 6th. Recognizing that Wendee would go mad waiting at home for the baby to come, Jane doesn't contradict those plans, but tries to temper them.

This cozy visit takes place at Wendee and Peter's. A circular quilt-covered bed is currently the centrepiece of their living room, because the bedroom is being painted. This is convenient for Wendee's physical check-up, and also presents an almost irresistable birthing environment, everyone admits. This will be their labouring place. But Wendee privately reveals that she is willing to have a hospital birth ''as a gift to Peter this time.'' This expression of her love has clearly touched him. He cuddles Wendee, jokes with a new ease, and declares that the baby recognizes his voice these days.

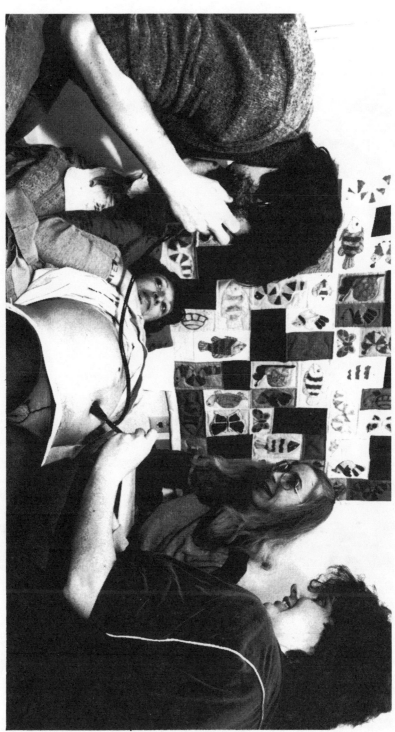

Peter listens to his baby.

E. Barrington

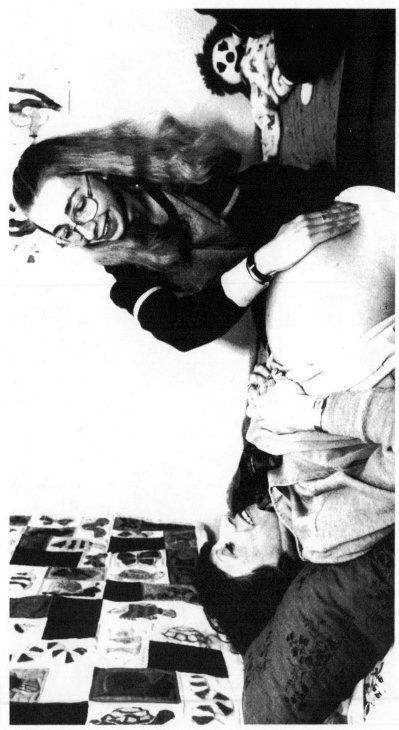

Midwife Jane palpates Wendee's baby.

Wendee describes the new sensations of her last few days. Wednesday evening she worked till midnight and the baby made her pay:

> I was all aches. We were stuffing pillows everywhere and that didn't help. Then last night, I have a feeling the baby dropped. I feel more pressure down here. Is that it?

Perhaps the baby is a *little* closer to being engaged in Wendee's pelvis, Jane affirms when she palpates, but it is still fairly high and *very* active. Wendee has taken to propping herself up on pillows so she can watch the action in her own full-bloomed belly.

The next visit — perhaps the last? — is back at Jane's on Friday.

Labour Commences — Early hours, Tuesday, March 27th. 38 1/2 weeks.

Wakened by contractions in the night, Wendee waits till 7:30 a.m. to call Jane. Her midwife keeps her on the phone for two contractions, noting that Wendee is still able to talk through them. Jane decides she has time to take Parrish to daycare before heading over to check Wendee's dilation.

Although Wendee has had contractions for several hours, she is only one centimeter dilated. Jane advises her to eat, rest between contractions, and keep in touch. She should conserve energy, because it could be a long haul.

Wendee cancels her business appointments, but she and Peter spend much of the day doing errands and "getting things ready." When Jane calls mid-afternoon Wendee is about to take a nap. The contractions have spaced further apart. On Tuesday night she is able to get some sleep between them.

At 9:00 a.m. Wednesday Jane comes and discovers Wendee is still only at three centimeters. Contractions are following a strong-weak-weak pattern. The midwife orders her client in mock sterness to eat breakfast. She'll need the food energy for the duration.

Peter declares at this point that he feels comfortable about staying home for the birth. The "impasse" between the couple that has marked most of their pregnancy has conveniently dissolved at the crucial moment. Both partners have generously deferred to the other's wishes. Now anything can happen. Jane is pleased.

Returning at 1:00 p.m. Jane finds Wendee and Peter somewhat discouraged at the slow pace of their labour. She suggests a leisurely walk, and offers to wait for them at home.

When they return, midwife and parents watch the movie *Flashdance* on the video equipment they rented to film the birth. Wendee turns the sound off during heavy contractions. Jane checks her again at 4:30 p.m. and discovers she's up to five centimeters. Theo arrives shortly afterward and the couple are buoyed by their midwives' sense of progress.

Sometimes Wendee paces the length of the room between contractions; sometimes she sits on the diaper-covered couch, or sprawls on the bed. Peter is intensely focussed on her needs, shifting to support her weight when she squats to get the most out of every contraction. "They're madly in love," Jane observes approvingly.

Vital signs remain strong. Wendee still gets rests between contractions, and in spite of the long hours of labour, copes admirably with her pains. She blows away the tension each time, and never complains above a moan, though Jane encourages her to make noise. Theo remains a vigilant presence, offering only occasional encouragement.

At 11:00 p.m., after almost 48 hours of labour, Jane masks her disappointment at finding Wendee only six to seven centimeters dilated. The bag of waters has not broken and without the pressure of the baby's head on the cervix, dilation could continue at this slow pace for too many hours. Contractions still haven't assumed a hard and fast pattern, so Jane offers Wendee a natural homeopathic tincture, caullophyllum, which may strengthen the contractions.

Because Wendee has heartburn and hasn't eaten much since breakfast, Jane is not surprised to find ketones in her urine. This is a sign of physical exhaustion. Yet in spite of the stress on her body that the ketonuria indicates, Wendee continues to walk about, even climb stairs to the bathroom. She looks merely exhausted instead of faint. Her endurance is remarkable.

Jane prescribes a banana yoghurt smoothie for fast energy. Wendee dutifully sips it down. Eyes propped open, Peter continues to support his wife through every move of her labour.

At 2:00 a.m. Jane and Theo check Wendee and assess the situation. She is barely seven centimeters and the baby is still too active to engage in her pelvis. Wendee should not labour much longer or she'll be too physically exhausted to push at second stage. In conference with Wendee and Peter, they decide it would be appropriate to move to hospital. There, Wendee's waters could be broken without the small risk of cord prolapse. She could have a glucose I.V. to boost her energy. Jane calls Wendee's doctor. This is no emergency, but a cautious choice the midwives make, aware of Peter's predisposition toward hospital birth.

Slowly, Wendee is coddled into the car. Theo calls out encouragement as she heads for home. The transfer to Toronto General Hospital is smoothly accomplished by 3:00 a.m.

The nurse who receives them is cheerful and cooperative. She permits the entire support team into the birthing room (Jane, Peter and I are all allowed to stay by her side).

The resident breaks the waters, but ever-vigilant, Wendee refuses to allow an internal fetal heart monitor. "No! No medical intervention," she declares between contractions. The resident shrugs and the nurse sets up an external monitor for just twenty minutes. An acceptable compromise, says Jane. Baby is still strong and Wendee's contractions gain force.

Around 6:00 a.m., when Wendee is beginning to despair, she finally hits full dilation and is gripped by a powerful urge to push. She bursts into the first tears of this prolonged labour; and then somehow summons her determination to push her baby out. Jane lauds her efforts, croons encouragement. Midwife and husband hold Wendee's hands.

The obstetrician arrives and after only a half hour of pushing, baby's head shows at Wendee's perineum. Jane guides Wendee's hand down to touch her baby's head. Recognition flashes across this mother's face and she pushes with renewed vigour. She shouts with the burning sensation of her stretching perineum. The doctor stands back, allowing Wendee to proceed naturally. Perhaps too naturally! He does not adequately support her perineum as the baby's head suddenly emerges. A sharp cry from Wendee as a big shoulder pops out, and she tears.

But never mind, she doesn't feel the wound. Here is a baby. A baby the doctor tenderly transfers to Wendee's chest. "It's a boy," Peter whispers to her. "Sean," Wendee sighs tentatively to her new infant. Nobody is tired anymore. No one disturbs the romance of the new family. Wendee and Peter are oblivious to all but the new being, enthusiastically sucking at her breast minutes after its birth. (Wendee barely notices the doctor suturing her second-degree tear.) 6:37 a.m. Thursday, March 29th, 1984. Sean Nasmith. Weighing in at 8 1/2 pounds. A champagne welcome. Jane beams with pride.

Four hours later, after a pediatrician checks Sean, Jane sees the new family home. They sign themselves out of the hospital in favour of their own family bed. Three fall asleep in each others' arms.

Postpartum Visit #1 — Friday, March 30.

> Wendee is a very healthy woman, and she is simply too efficient to
> bleed!
>
> — Jane

Such is Wendee's stamina that she actually answered the doorbell a half
hour after the family fell asleep on the birthday. The hydro meter reader
was astounded when she apologized for taking so long, declaring that
she'd just had a baby. "This morning?" he exclaimed in disbelief.
"Here?!" "Sort of," Wendee replied.

Parents and midwife barely have energy to laugh at this story on the
first postpartum visit, but Wendee is doing fine physically. Peter looks
like it is he who has survived an ordeal. Luckily, the overactive young
Sean finally decided to sleep the day he was born and didn't demand a
feed till 5:00 p.m.

Jane checks Wendee's breasts, pulse and blood pressure. (See Chart
page 81.) She suggests sitz baths in epsom salts, comfrey and garlic to
heal the stitches on her perineum.

Then she gives Sean a thorough newborn exam. Concerned about a
retracted breathing pattern, she suggests Wendee and Peter take him to
a pediatrician for a second look. (They make a visit to Sick Children's
Hospital that afternoon and are told it's not a problem.) He is feeding
well and appears to have Wendee's physical resiliency.

Wendee and Peter will move to her parents' house today, where they
can be looked after for awhile.

Postpartum Visit #2 — Saturday, March 31st.

> So you're Jane? I've heard so much good about you, I expected to
> see a halo!
>
> — Cecil Wood, Wendee's father

Wendee greets Jane at the door of the Woods' house, dressed, made up,
hair curled. Already she has learned how to breastfeed standing up and
appears to be full of energy. Her milk is coming in and aside from the
sore stitches, she has no problems to report. But she fires questions at
Jane every few minutes, while Peter beams on her and proud grand-
parents hover about. "How long will I take to heal?" "How do you tell
when the milk is in?" "I can feel contractions in my stomach when he
feeds. How long will that go on?"

Sean sleeps peacefully, failing to wake even when Jane checks him
over. He is wetting the expected ten diapers a day, Wendee reports, and
sleeping with her or Peter quite contentedly at night.

POSTPARTUM CARE RECORD

VISIT #1   DATE: _Mar 30/84_   heart rate 120;

baby: nursing well, mild heat rash, cord fine, reflexes good
      breathing a txt labored w/some chest retractions
      (advised to see pediatrician today) good strong cry

Wendee: BP 105/65 temp 36.5 stitches look fine, breasts fine
        pulse 64. looking & feeling great.

VISIT #2   DATE: _Mar 31/84_

baby: nursing well, still sleeping lots, cord fine
      breathing fine now - was checked out at Sick Kids

Wendee: BP 110/70 pulse 60, milk coming in
        doing fine, flow light, stitches
        healing

VISIT #3   DATE: _Apr 1/84_

Baby: no noticable jaundice, has nursed a bunch
      today

Wendee: tired, doing fine, pulse 60
        lots of milk, stitches fine

VISIT #4   DATE: _Apr 2/84_

Theo did visit
        Baby gassy, fussy. Wendee tired

VISIT #5   DATE: _Apr 3/84_

Baby: burping is helping gas, cord looks good.
      has gained 12lb. did PKU.

Wendee: stitches, uterus fine, first b.m. since birth
        100/65 pulse 60 doing very well

VISIT #6   DATE: _____

CHECK THE FOLLOWING:

The Mother:
Breasts and nipples
Perineum
Uterus
Lochia
Temperature
Pulse
Haemoglobin (when
            needed)

The Baby:
Heart & Lungs
Cord
Head
Diaper area
Rashes
Nursing
Jaundice
General appearance
Temperment
Reflexes

Please notify the
primary midwife if
you notice anything
out of the ordinary.

Name of mother:
Wendee Wood
Date of birth:
March 29, 1984

Discussion moves back to the labour and birth, reliving details and comparing perspectives. Then to the new parenthood. They have made a video of the first diaper change. A comedy, Peter promises.

Jane answers questions in detail, examines Wendee and emphasizes that a new mother needs rest: "Your body is going through the hormone changes of nine months, in reverse, in two weeks. Pace yourself. Watch out for 'end of the first week wipe-out!'"

Postpartum Visit #3 — Sunday, April 1.

> I really appreciate your sensitivity to where the two of us were coming from, Jane. I think you chose right in suggesting we go to hospital. I thought you were reading us both very well.
>
> — Wendee

Wendee is admitting to feeling tired by day four, but she is healing well and her uterus is shrinking neatly, Jane observes. Her milk has arrived in full flow, and Sean shows no sign of even normal physiologic jaundice, so common among newborns. For all of their arduous labour, these new parents are being blessed with an easy postpartum — so far.

Postpartum Visit #4 — Monday, April 2nd.

> If he has gassy episodes, look back at what you've been eating. Some babies react if you drink lots of cow's milk, or eat anything from the cabbage family.
>
> — Theo

Sean is gorging himself on the new milk, Wendee reports to Theo, who comes to make this visit. He drinks so much he spits up, and then is fussy with gas.

After checking Wendee's stitches and approving their healing, Theo concentrates on gas remedies. She shows Wendee ways of burping Sean, and positions to hold him in to release the gas.

Wendee admits that her son's discomfort has been very demanding. "He had me run ragged. I finally just handed him over to Peter last night."

Postpartum Visit #5 — Tuesday, April 3rd.

> At some point when you're about to get up and do something because someone else is holding the baby, say to yourself, "No. I'll do some exercises instead."
>
> — Jane

Although Wendee looks forward to getting back to her yoga, she isn't finding time yet to do the exercises she needs for her uterus and tummy muscles. Even the sitz baths are hard to fit into her full days.

On this last visit of the series, Jane does the obligatory PKU test, unpleasant but necessary. Pricking an indignant Sean's heel to draw blood, Jane makes sure that grandmother's and mother's arms offer comfort. Unfortunately, Sean's blood is clotting so effectively that it's difficult to squeeze out enough. But finally it is done. Jane carries the test package to the post office immediately after the visit.

Wendee elicits Jane's advice about a pediatrician for Sean, and asks specific questions about her newborn's development: "How far can he focus now?" "From your breast to your face," Jane answers.

They talk about burping and breastfeeding techniques, and about Wendee and Peter's travel plans for the following month. Parents, baby and both "woofs" will slowly caravan back and forth across the country in a camper trailer, aiming to visit two great-grandparents on the West Coast and one on the East. Knowing Wendee, this ambition is not impossible.

On April 27th, just before they leave, Jane promises a final postpartum appointment to discuss birth control and any parenting problems. She can fit Wendee with a diaphragm or cervical cap then, if she wants. The midwife also has advice on travelling with an infant. Jane actually discovered a way to breastfeed Parrish in his backwards infant car seat. Wendee looks forward to this.

With hugs and copious thanks, Wendee lets Jane go. "Just because the visits are over doesn't mean you can't call," Jane reminds over her shoulder.

"I know," Wendee responds confidently. Jane is *involved* with them. She'll be "on call" as long as this new family needs her. And they love her for it.

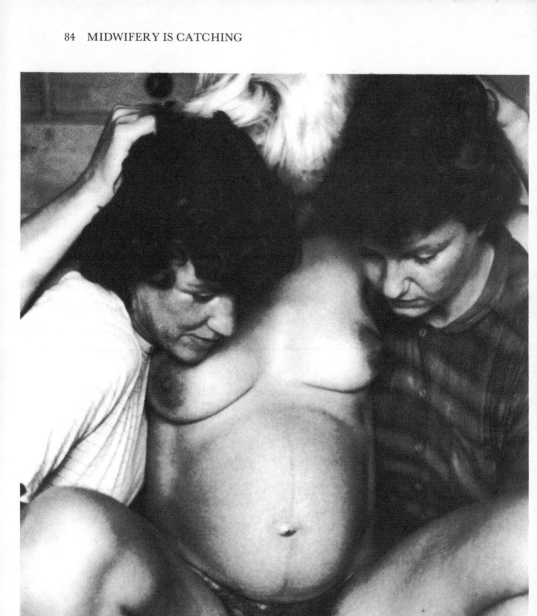

Midwife Sue Rose and friend Janet support Joe as her baby's head crowns.

Chapter Six
Portraits of Practice

Community Midwifery

Midwifery always takes on local colours. Although the rise of the new midwifery was a continent-wide phenomenon of the 1970s, it was also a grassroots community response to local needs. It flourished only where parents perceived some lack in the available maternity care system; only where women of the community were willing to take on the responsibilities of birth work.

The greatest strength, and perhaps the most intriguing aspect of midwifery, is its ability to respond to particular needs. A clientele of ethnic mothers in the inner city elicits a different style of care than the women of a rural spiritual community. Actions and attitudes essential to one midwife's practice might be utterly inappropriate in another's setting. When midwives get together there are always exclamations of amazement about how each other works. Yet they share a fundamentally similar philosophy.

The factors that provoke the emergence of midwifery in a given community and then tailor its ways vary widely from coast to coast. Sometimes the impetus is philosophical, political or spiritual, a strain of ideas or beliefs common among the populace. Sometimes it is a traditional or cultural framework that fits a midwife into her place. Sometimes geography creates a practical necessity, or hospital policy provokes opposition and alternative.

In a city like Toronto, several different practices respond to particular groups. They cater to modesty-conscious ethnic minorities, consumer-conscious professionals, feminists, and the family-centred mothering movement. In a more homogeneous district, one dominant cultural stream might float a midwifery practice.

Across the country a score of different midwifery styles highlight the values of their client community, reflecting local cultures or sub-cultures, as well as individual midwives' personalities. By way of illustration, I describe two rather extraordinary midwifery practices I visited in the Fall of 1983. Both are small-town/rural in orientation. But what else do they have in common?

The Old Order Mennonite practice in the Waterloo, Ontario district, and the new-age community in the Kootenay mountains of British Columbia are two distinctive examples of how midwifery care moulds to meet unusual cultural and community needs. Each exemplifies the responsiveness that is essential to the art of midwifery.

Midwifery in the Kootenays: "Community Ties that Bond"

> I live in this community with these people. We've taken on this life-style of changes. We're committed to a much greater thing than home birth. It's much bigger than I realized myself. We *need* each other.
>
> — Pat Armstrong, R.N.

Pat Armstrong, the first of the new midwives to practise in the Kootenay Region of British Columbia, speaks of the commitment in her community with real urgency. "Community" here connotes more than mere physical proximity. It means "intentional community" and "alternative community" with all the attendant ideals. Commitment means sharing, the operative principles that ensures the community's growth.

Since the 1960s, thousands of determined young idealists from across the continent have drawn together in the Kootenay mountain district. Along the Nelson River system and up the Slocan Valley, the back-to-nature "hippies" cleared land for their ongoing life experiment. From New York City and Nova Scotia they arrived in search of independence. They wanted to learn what self-sufficiency might grow from an intimate connection with nature. They chose to practice cooperation, without the fetters of regulation. This "Kootenay new-age community" did social pioneering. Midwifery became an important part of it.

Both the geography and ideology of the Kootenays demanded the alternative of home birth. Many home-steading women were simply too isolated up winding mountain roads to make it to the hospital on time. Others, according to a physician in the local town of New Denver, found hospital birth "contrary to their lifestyle, desires and family functioning. Their whole being rejects what is offered in hospital."

Disillusioned with the limitations of middle-class family life, the Kootenay folk hoped to forge new relationships with their children. And they were willing to begin before birth. Back in the sixties, young couples were talking about "total caring" for babies' physical, psycho-emotional and spiritual needs. Newborn sensitivity and awareness were widely acknowledged here. The term "bonding" had not yet been coined, but these families sought "togetherness." Along with concepts like "the family bed," and the eventuality of home schooling, a sensitive, family-centred home birth made sense to them.

Perhaps one quarter of the total population of Nelson and environs in the 1970s was new-age immigrants. Consequently the Selkirk Health District (centred in Nelson), developed the highest proportion of home births in British Columbia, perhaps all of Canada. A study produced for Health and Welfare Canada in 1980 showed that in the late 1970s, close to eight percent of births in Selkirk District occurred at home, whereas in most districts it accounts for only 1-2 percent. Many more Kootenay parents desired a home birth, and everyone at least knew someone who had given birth at home.

During the years covered by that study, 1977-80, most of the home births were attended by the midwives of the Kootenay Childbirth Counselling Centre, or Dr. Carolyn deMarco, who worked cooperatively with them. The beginnings of home birth locally, however, go back to the late 1960s. Committed independantistes began choosing not to go to hospital, even if that meant "going it alone" at home. There were few other options until Pat Armstrong arrived.

Armstrong, a nurse, arrived with her family in the Slocan Valley to build a new life and a new home in 1970, when she was 30. They came from California, where she had trained as a Lamaze teacher and studied with gynaecologists at Stanford University. Pat set up childbirth classes in the Slocan in 1971.

A couple in her first class declared that they were preparing to do their own birth at home. Pat grew close to the woman as the classes progressed, so she agreed to help out at the birth. She had been to a few births in California, and exchanged home birth research with midwife Raven Lang. But Pat was most definitely not a midwife — yet.

> That birth was a remarkable experience. Those people were younger than me but I had been living down the middle of the road, and they had been investigating different ways of thinking and being. They understood the risks in their birth and saw their responsibility.
>
> They grasped that we are required to take responsibility to make changes in our society and ourselves. That means risk — not safety risk, not foolish risk, but what you might call courage.
>
> I knew some technical stuff — more than I had thought — but those people taught me how to have faith and manage a birth. They were my teachers, my inspiration.
>
> After that, going to births, I just kept learning *big things*, about living and what people can do.

Working on her own, Pat attended an average of two home births a month for the next couple of years. She gradually took on more responsibility, and studied how to cope with possible complications. She noticed that the parents, too, grew more intense about their birth preparations.

The fathers became more actively involved, not just with birth, but with their infant offspring.

Always cautious lest there be postpartum hemorrhage or illness in the newborn, Pat generally stayed for three days around a birth. Some people didn't have telephones and she wasn't comfortable 30 miles down a mountain road away from a new mother.

Her "practice," an informal service for friends and neighbours, grew to four births a month. By 1974, the physical and emotional demands began to exhaust her. In response to her own needs and those of her five children, she began to move back into nursing. Over the next few years she eased out of midwifery, attending only a few friends' births.

Pat caught about a hundred babies at home in the Kootenays before she turned her attention to reforming hospital birth practices. It is said that at Slocan Community Hospital, the ten-bed unit where she now works, you can have a hospital birth almost as nice as home.

In Fall of 1974, just as Pat was slowing down, Camille Bush came to Nelson. A 24-year-old mother who had apprenticed in midwifery at the Vancouver Birth Centre earlier that year, Camille was drawn to the Kootenays by the evidence of a true cooperative lifestyle. A job opening for a health worker at the Nelson Women's Centre convinced her that she was indeed in the right place.

Pat Armstrong referred some pregnant women to the new midwife in town, and Camille began attending the occasional birth. She set up alternative (to the Public Health Department) childbirth education classes at the Women's Centre. Camille carefully avoided the word "midwife" in those days, lest it frighten some women away from the Centre. Even at births, she was most comfortable with the role of "facilitator," aiding the parents in their undertaking.

Home birth parents in the isolated circumstances of the Kootenays had to be especially well motivated, and highly self-sufficient. They read extensively and prepared psychologically. One woman drove 75 miles into Nelson for every prenatal class and clinic. There were very few emergencies in Camille's early years of practice, a fact that she attributes to the rigourous self-selection process for home birth.

The pioneering "back-to-the-land" women who comprised much of her clientele were in fine physical shape. They ate out of their organic gardens, chopped firewood, and helped build their own homes. A Kootenay woman wouldn't necessarily shy away from shingling a roof at seven months pregnant.

Men and women alike did back-breaking seasonal labour on tree-planting crews. One mother who'd been known to plant two thousand trees in a day, was actually able to jog right through all her contractions. Then she climbed up a ladder into her house at full dilation. So there was no need to encourage "exercise" at prenatal classes in Nelson. And in ten years of practise, Camille encountered only three cigarette smokers.

Dr. Carolyn deMarco came to the Kootenays shortly after Camille, and set up a general practice in Slocan City. Carolyn had seen one hundred births during her internship at Toronto East General Hospital. One was a natural birth, and it had impressed her. She read midwife Raven Lang's *Birth Book* while travelling across the country, and determined to do home births when she settled in the valley.

Carolyn called Pat Armstrong for advice before she attended her first home birth. What equipment should she carry? The list was simple then: items like hemostats, scissors, and dental floss or the traditional sterile shoelace, to tie the cord. That list was to grow more complex each year.

Carolyn found her first few home births harrowing, even with a friend coaching her through the unfamiliar routine. "After the birth everybody would be sitting upstairs drinking champagne, and I'd be sitting downstairs by myself, worrying about every possible complication." Her doctor's training had not inspired faith in nature. "Nature will tear the woman apart!" an obstetrician had once assured her.

Before the next birth she called Camille, who was also still somewhat uneasy about attending alone. They decided to see women together. Camille shared her experience with natural home birth, and Carolyn contributed her Gestalt psychology training. The physician found studies in psycho-emotional areas a greater asset than her medical background. She felt that the amount of medical technology she could carry around wouldn't make the crucial difference.

The home birthing community around Nelson was ready to work with her psychological tools. They comprehended the body-mind connection and wanted to deal with labour on *all* its levels. The Kootenay Childbirth Counselling Centre used visualization techniques long before such methods were validated by the medical research of Gayle Peterson and Louis Mehl, M.D.

Although Carolyn usually called herself a midwife during the 1970s, and the birth attendants worked as equals, the weight of legal responsibility inevitably fell to her, because of her credentials. With an M.D. on the scene, the self-selection process for home birth parents slackened. It became an option for couples who would never have thought to "go it alone."

A lawyer advised Carolyn to have parents sign informed consents, accepting their own responsibility for the birth outcome. She and Camille developed a home birth screening process that explored beyond mere physical contra-indications for home birth like breech positions, twins, and pregnancy complications. They required parents to attend prenatal classes and clinics, make specific preparations for birth, and demonstrate a real ability to adapt to the demands of pregnancy.

One further requirement for home birth, addressed to a population that drove jalopies on treacherous mountain roads, was typed in block letters across the bottom of their prenatal forms. "Do you have a vehicle THAT CAN BE RELIED ON in case of transfer to hospital?"

By 1976, Barb Ray and Abra Palumbo were welcomed into the practice as apprentices. Barb had experienced a natural birth at home in the Kootenays in 1975, despite a previous cesarean section. Abra had gone all the way to Alaska five years earlier to find a native midwife for her first home birth. With two more midwives on the team it was finally practical for the Kootenay midwives to attend labours in pairs. They arranged the luxury of a third woman for back-up.

All the midwives were involved in prenatal clinics, day-long affairs at Carolyn's house every second Sunday. As well as their physical check-ups, women shared experiences with other home birthers. There were regular discussion groups for parents with visiting speakers. Lunch and babysitting were provided. For all this, people paid two dollars. *If* they could afford it.

The services of a midwife for a home birth, including pre and postpartum visits, cost fifty to seventy-five dollars then. As members of a community that operated on minimal cash, the midwives were committed to remaining accessible to all who sought home birth. Sometimes that meant fees were paid in carpentry or garden vegetables. Camille was paid for one birth with a fresh-baked loaf of bread. Midwifery rarely covered its own costs.

In 1977, the local home birth boom began, and Camille left her job at the Women's Centre for full-time midwifery. She was involved with over 40 home births that year.

The Kootenay folk, living in their handcrafted homes (some with, and some without, electricity and running water), had by then developed their own traditions around childbirth. Since Pat Armstrong's early birthing days, neighbours always stocked a woman's freezer before her due date. Or casseroles would miraculously appear on the doorstep for three days postpartum.

Mothers and midwives got together to create the "Quilts of the Kootenays" to wrap the arriving infants. Each woman contributed a square depicting her message to mother and child. The quilt Camille Bush received for her first son Bryn in 1979 has a suede fetus in one corner, crafted by fellow midwife Abra Palumbo. In another patch is an embroidered biblical promise from a devout young Christian mother.

The naming of a child might take place any time from early pregnancy to weeks postpartum. It awaited some inspiration to the parents. "You don't go through all the changes involved in having a home birth and just call your child John," laughs Pat Armstrong. The Kootenay Valley has its Moses Moonshine and its Reuben Raphael, and then there are the siblings Sky, Shoshoni, Sundance and Starchild.

The "Blessing Way" ceremony, an adaptation of a Navajo Indian puberty rite, is often enacted prior to birth. Enthroned amidst cushions and flowers in a circle of singing and dancing friends, the honoured parents receive healing wishes and meaningful gifts. This rite of passage unfolds creatively according to the needs of the particular parents. Abra tells of one Blessing Way that evolved into a wedding.

Burial of the placenta or after-birth is ceremoniously observed here. But due to the frozen ground in winter, many a placenta spends a season in the freezer. Come spring planting time, it nurtures the roots of a new tree.

Occasionally, parents might choose to eat the placenta. (The hormones in it are helpful in preventing postpartum hemorrhage.) Camille Bush, a vegetarian for seven years at that time, recalls being handed a small bowl of placenta and vegetable stew after a birth. "I really went for the potatoes and carrots!" she laughs.

The rites and rituals around birth are as different as the families who create them. Children take on roles like community herald or time-keeper, announcing the moment of birth. The midwives go a long way to accomodate parents' particular wishes.

Ilene Bell, a Toronto midwife who landed in Nelson by accident in 1981, and stayed, recalls a birth "that could only have happened in the Kootenays." She attended it along with a former Toronto colleague, Judi Pustil, who joined her in Nelson in 1982.

A shy young couple living on a farm in Fruitvale, 30 miles south of Nelson, was expecting their third, and probably last child. They reveal-ed to Ilene a dream of an outdoor birth. That would have been fine, except that this baby was due in March. Ilene and Judi listened in amazement to the scenario the parents had devised.

The birth was to take place in a huge tent on a hillside. The couple had lived in the tent when they first moved onto her parents' farm, so it felt like home. They assured Ilene that, with the wood stove stoked, it would be warm enough.

Somewhat against their better judgement, she and Judi agreed. Ilene reasons that "ritualistic details are important. They make people feel secure, though they have nothing rational to do with safety."

The birth took place on a starry cold midnight, in the tent that proved to be *too* warm. The mother chose to deliver on hands and knees, so Ilene caught the baby virtually standing on her head on a grassy slope. Then she proceeded to suture a small tear by lantern light.

The event was topped off by a comical moonlit procession back down to the house. The father bundled his baby in his arms, and grandfather and uncle appeared with a wheelbarrow to transport the mother down the hill. To Ilene's amazement, the woman barely bled. The midwives laughed with nervous relief all the way home.

Like all the earlier Kootenay emigrés, Ilene and Judi grew into the community. They adapted to practices different from Toronto, where even midwifery moves faster.

In the Kootenays, there is more time to spend with each mother. Prenatal visits last at least an hour, and a home visit 40 miles from town inevitably stretches into an afternoon. Mothers' and midwives' lives intertwine. The sympathetic bond can grow so strong that a midwife experiences contractions along with a woman in labour.

Having a rural practice spread out across hundreds of square miles also affected the styles of Toronto midwives. Racing out to a precipitous birth there were no more red lights to worry about, but there were avalanches and mudslides. And it was a long ride to hospital in case of an emergency transfer.

Ilene missed the security of hospital support she had known in Toronto. In the mid-seventies nurses had come to the Women's Centre to sit in on Camille's childbirth classes. Midwives were allowed to accompany clients who had to be moved into hospital. Camille actually caught a client's baby in hospital, at a doctor's invitation. He even apologized that there was no olive oil for perineal massage.

But by the time Ilene arrived, hospital politics had changed to suit the times. Supportive physicians had moved on, and conservatism had moved in. In September 1982, a nurse who allowed one of the midwives into the labour room with a client was forbidden to do so again — unless she wanted to find work elsewhere.

This unwritten policy was not based on birth statistics. After over four hundred births, Pat and the Kootenay Childbirth Counselling Centre did not have a death until 1983. Even then, the stillbirth was due to multiple congenital heart defects, incompatible with life, and beyond any practitioner's hand.

There *were* some close calls. Ilene and Carolyn rescued a mother who suddenly began to bleed two weeks after her baby was born. They had to transport her by toboggan down a half-mile driveway, hip deep in snow. But they made it. Pat was once forced by emergency circumstances to attend a four-week premature home labour. It turned out to be surprise twins. She pumped breath into a three-pound lifeless baby, and coped with a severe maternal hemorrhage till she got the trio to hospital. The midwives had to be prepared not only to welcome life, but to turn death away.

The midwives of the Kootenay community participate in the full circle of life. Old clients call on them when the children are sick, or for support when a relative dies. Midwives meet mothers daily in the shopping centres, and they see the children they birthed growing up and going to school. They are drawn into many community decisions, as "wise women" and advisors.

Pat Armstrong muses about how she was reluctant to take the title "midwife" for several years after she began birth work. She was not ready to accept the weight of responsibility to the whole community that the midwife's role included. In the context of the Nelson new-age experiment, a midwife is guardian not just to the birth of a baby, but to the birth of a new sort of society. "Birthing is an important way of pioneering here," she explains, "and 'midwife' means a way of life."

Midwifery among the Mennonites: "Birth In Biblical Simplicity"

When I passed by thee
and saw thee polluted in thine own blood
I said unto thee
when thou wast in thy blood,
live.

— Ezekiel 16:6

"Now I'm not superstitious," Violet Ropp clarifies as she points out this biblical passage on the face page of her midwifery notebook, "but there *is* power in prayer."

Violet inherited the quotation from a former midwife in Southwestern Ontario, whose experiences attested to the power of the prayer. The midwife is locally renowned because her presence at births seemed to prevent maternal hemorrhage. When a baffled physician finally enquired about her technique, the wise woman answered with Ezekiel 16:6, "I pray."

The Bible is the dominant symbol among the Old Order Mennonite and Amish people whom Violet and her partner Elsie Cressman feel privileged to serve as midwives. But Elsie and Violet do not simply rely on prayer to ensure the outcome of births they attend. Both are Registered Nurses with Bachelor's degrees and British midwifery training, and they contend that experience with normal birth is their greatest asset.

Elsie Cressman is a stout energetic woman of Waterloo region farming stock. She remained single, to adventure as a nurse with the Mennonite Mission in Africa for 22 years. In 1970, between stints in Somalia and Kenya, Elsie took a sabbatical to study midwifery in England. By the time she returned home to Kitchener in 1976 she had seen one thousand births.

In spite of being over 60 and having a heart problem, Elsie was not ready to retire. She took up nursing at St. Mary's Hospital but soon that was not occupation enough. When she got wind of lay midwives Willy Mattocks and Mary Molnar practising in town, she too began to answer young couples' determined calls for home births.

In 1980 Elsie met Violet Ropp, fellow Conference Mennonite, missionary nurse, and British-trained midwife; the ideal complement to her particular style of practice. Elsie admits she dragged then 39-year-old Violet into an apprenticeship-cum-partnership, the younger woman all the while protesting that the duties of farmwife and mother were workload enough.

But Violet did protest too much. Since she watched her sister born from her crib in the bedroom corner, birth has been in Violet's blood. In her twenties, this romantic missionary nurse was wooed by one-room cabin births in the Northern Ontario Indian village of Tikkangikum. Midwifery finally won her in 1974, when the doors opened to allow her the long-cherished year of training in England.

Her marriage to a Mennonite farmer followed midwifery certification almost immediately, and Violet's next experience with birth was personal. There was the brief life of an anencephalic son in 1977, and then the disappointment of repeat cesareans for Hubert and Rudy in 1978 and 1980. Having endured the anguish of unsatisfying, unsupported births, Violet was evermore determined to offer other women undivided attention for every contraction. The final stage of her apprenticeship only awaited Elsie Cressman's urgings.

Violet brought to the midwifery partnership an instinctive talent for relaxing labouring women. Elsie added a rare confidence and expertise, accumulated over the years in Africa. There are differences and disagreements between these women, but while presiding at births, they melt wordlessly into the common cause. "We get so intertwined," Elsie remarks proudly, "that the woman doesn't always know who delivered."

Violet and Elsie both belong to a strain of conservative Mennonites that looks liberal when compared to their Old Order clientele. The two midwives assimilate easily into small town Ontario culture. They appreciate all the modern amenities. The only immediate evidence of their religion is the pleated white net cap covering a graying bun on the back of each midwife's head. Elsie and Violet wear these "prayer coverings" everywhere. Old Order women even wear them when they're in labour.

Various splinter churches of the Old Order Mennonite and Amish co-exist in the Kitchener-Waterloo area. Elsie and Violet had to learn to distinguish their different sensibilities. It seems that there are many interpretations of the Biblical command to be "in the world but not of it." While Old Order households reject telephones, electricity, automobiles and indoor plumbing, here and there a curious compromise crops up. There is a telephone box at the roadside of a horse-and-buggy lane. There is the buggy man who drives a truck in town by day.

Invited into an Old Order kitchen, the visitor feels distinctly *out* of this world. Wood stove, wash stand, straight-back wooden chairs. Kindly hostess Louisa is clad in an ankle-length workdress and kerchief. Unlike the pioneer village performers she evokes, Louisa defers very real chores to sit down and talk with her midwife.

She belongs to the most conservative faction of the Old Order Mennonites, and — perhaps not so surprisingly — she was the first to appeal to the midwives for a home birth. "Christians will seek to maintain simplicity in all areas of life," their teachings say. Auto trips to hospital and medical technology were difficult for Louisa to reconcile with that "simplicity."

Mennonite values and medical technology are such an obvious culture clash that it is shocking to discover no active midwives among the Old Order themselves. Since midway through the childbearing years of the "grandmother generation," Old Order babies have been born in hospital. The reason is simple. The doctors stopped coming out to the farms. Women were told they must go to hospital to birth safely, and Mennonites do not question authority. Not even medical authority.

Louisa tells her story in a unique English, influenced by the Bible and accented with the Pennsylvania Dutch they speak among themselves. She was 27, and pregnant with her second child, when she read about Elsie Cressman in the *Elmira Signal*. She wrote a note to the midwife, revealing her desire "since maidenhood" to have her babies at home. Her letter was an act of radical conservatism. She broke from the norm to enhance her Old Order values.

The doctor in town received his Mennonite patient's home birth plans with horror. "Why wait nine months for a dead baby?" he asked her. Ever tactful, Louisa let him talk.

"I wrote to Elsie looking for advice and help and encouragement," Louisa declares. "And that's what I got. I don't know what we'd have done if we couldn't get her." She hesitates, then speculates that "maybe we'd have done it alone." Some of her Old Order neighbours had recently taken to doing just that.

Some of Louisa's reasons for choosing a midwife-attended home birth sound strikingly like those of her liberated city sisters. Others are distinct to her spiritual culture. "The hospital is a grand modern place," Louisa admires, "but I was afraid I wouldn't have my thoughts thankful enough towards God, being in such a different place."

A neighbour expresses their cultural concern for propriety. "Why, at the hospital, they say we're to leave our modesty at the door, and pick it up on our way out," she repeats indignantly.

Elsie huffs that it is the ultimate indignity — and utterly unsafe — when these women give birth en route to hospital. It is not an uncommon experience, given the short labours for seventh or tenth babies, and the distances of up to 60 miles to the city.

Mennonite men often cite transportation as their first reason for calling upon the midwives. When a woman goes into labour, it is her husband's duty to go wake up a non-Old Order neighbour to use the phone. He must call the doctor and the ambulance, or ask the farmer to drive them to the hospital. Meanwhile everyone wonders if they will make it on time. Or worse, will they arrive only to be turned around because the contractions have ceased?

"It isn't *only* because of the mileage," one home birth father felt the need to add, but he and others certainly appreciate the midwives coming to them. When Elsie is on duty at the hospital, Violet covers the practice. Help is only one call from the neighbour's.

Ironically, the midwives' only obstacle to birthing in these pioneer households is getting there. When winter storms blow snow across the country roads, arriving on time is a nerve-wracking touch and go. Otherwise, both women claim there's not much more to contend with than at any home birth. The midwives arrive with their instruments already sterilized. The husband hammers a big nail into the bedroom ceiling and hangs a lantern. And there's no secret to boiling water on a wood stove, says Elsie, who grew up doing just that.

The majority of these clients are having second or subsequent births. First babies are still born in hospital, in compliance with cautions from physicians and mothers-in-law. Young Mennonite home birth couples are ever respectful of the doctors, but they can't help but criticize hospitals. Their comments carry the same intent as those voiced by city folks, but these agricultural people colour their criticisms with barnyard metaphor.

"To my mind, the delivery room, with the doctor up on his high chair, why it looks like a slaughter house," declares one woman. "Stirrups are for horses, not for women," says another. One father wrote of the "rugged butcheryness" of his wife's first delivery in hospital, and another regretted seeing his dear wife "penned up in a farrowing room," like his pigs. "No wonder city men get nervous [about birth]," points out a barn-wise Mennonite father. "Why they've never seen anything being born!"

Louisa was the first of the Old Order to write to the midwives, citing some of these reasons for preferring a home birth. Soon her notes, offering "fond greetings of love and Remembrance this fine morning," were not the only ones arriving in the Cressman mailbox. Relying on Canada Post, and an even slower horse and buggy grapevine, Louisa's sister-in-law Lovina, and another relative Edna, sent the midwives their requests for a visit. All three women delivered inside of one week, Louisa's daughter Saloma coming last, on July 24, 1980.

Two months later, another relative, Minerva, gave birth at home, and soon a network of sisters and sisters-in-law was copying out Elsie's address for each other. In the first three years of practice, the midwives attended over 30 Old Order births, easily half of their home birth activity. Many Old Order families still choose hospital birth, where Elsie and Violet are not permitted to follow, yet their practice is growing fast.

Money is a factor in the choice of home birth for the Mennonites because they don't subscribe to socialized medicine. They will be beholden to no government, since they won't fight the government's wars. They pay taxes, but they will not even accept a Social Insurance Number. (That the S.I.N. acronym spells 'sin' has not escaped them.) When a Mennonite baby is born in hospital, the father or the church fund pays out perhaps $1500. The midwives' fee of $500 looks mild by comparison. Elsie appreciates that these Mennonite men always have their cheques ready.

Once the initial storm of reaction had passed, several of the local doctors, including the "nine months for a dead baby" optimist, began to cooperate with the midwives to back them up for Old Order home births. These physicians recognised that Elsie and Violet were offering services that a culturally isolated community lacked.

"The Mennonites are a neglected people," Elsie points out. Their women tend to see a doctor only once in the course of pregnancy, often at an advanced stage. Prenatal education was non-existent until the midwives began providing it door-to-door. The logistics of bringing pregnant couples from across the county together by horse and buggy for prenatal classes are absurd. Instead, Elsie and Violet clock hundreds of miles in their cars each week, making prenatal and postpartum visits from Wallenstein to Winterbourne to Wingham.

Perhaps because of the prenatal care, perhaps because their clients are so hearty, working well past the onset of labour, Elsie and Violet have yet to encounter a crisis requiring transport to hospital. What they do encounter is women like Nancy, who was in the kitchen preparing breakfast a half an hour before her baby was born. "She put out the good china and everything," exclaims Elsie, whose protests at the time were not heeded. The birth went well. And breakfast was delicious.

The only tragedy that has befallen this midwifery practice is Maple Syrup Urine Disease among the newborn. It is a hereditary intolerance to protein that circulates in the closed circles of Old Order genes. With second cousins marrying, it is not surprising that M.S.U.D. has claimed several of Elsie and Violet's babies. Even with intensive treatment at Sick Children's Hospital in Toronto, "maple syrup" children survive only months or years.

Although M.S.U.D. cannot be detected prenatally or prevented, the midwives make clear to their clients that many other perinatal problems can be avoided by appropriate medical action. They hand out books to read, insist that women see their doctors, and dispatch reluctant mothers to obstetricians at times.

One such case was a 34-year-old woman, determined to have her first child at home. The midwives only got wind of her at her 32nd week of pregnancy. By then she had high blood pressure and other symptoms of toxemia. Evidently, the woman was shocked to find herself pregnant by her 64-year-old, post-vasectomy husband, and she did not embrace the prospect of motherhood.

Cuddling her two-year-old daughter in her lap, that mother recalls appreciatively how the midwives sent her to her doctor. He "talked himself black and blue" trying to discourage her home birth plans. Then they dragged her to an obstetrician. Violent spent many hours on that farm, informally counselling, listening and sharing. By the time the baby was due — indeed welcome — all symptoms of toxemia had disappeared. The home birth plan was judged a safe bet after all.

Her jovial, gray-bearded Amish husband, already grandfather to 46, observed his daughter's birth from the daybed in their unlit kitchen, his interest disguised by the darkness. His love for the little girl born that December night is not disguised at all.

As the midwives' practice spread west into the Amish lands near Stratford, Elsie and Violet began to discover the fine distinctions between Old Order Amish and Mennonites. Aside from the obvious indicator of the Amish men's long beards, they learned that Amish fathers didn't attend births. The Mennonite men always assumed they'd be by their wives' sides in labour. Local doctors had allowed them in delivery rooms long before other fathers. But Violet found she had to assert her nursely authority to coax Amish men by the elbow to their own bedroom doors.

Except of course, for the Amish bishop who *really* got involved. His wife laboured only 90 minutes with their ninth child, and the baby beat Elsie. The midwives relayed telephone instructions just before the baby was born, and the father handily clamped and cut his daughter's cord.

The mother, who recalls sitting in the car holding back her previous baby till they made it to hospital, was thrilled with the home birth. She observes that her husband was immediately in love with the baby he caught, and with the next one, born at home of course. Well forewarned, Elsie and Violet arrived on time for the birth of this Amish couple's tenth babe.

Louisa and her husband Josiah were the midwives' first repeat couple. Shortly after their little Rebecca was born in November 1982, Elsie and Violet found themselves making rounds to other familiar households. But the midwives had successfully postponed what would have been annual repeat business by encouraging breastfeeding. It had been over two years since the last round of procreation among their couples.

This "natural spacing" of the family by breastfeeding was acceptable in a culture where birth control is verboten and children come from God. The midwives soon realized why the Old Order had gone over to bottles along with the rest of North America. These women had trouble finding time away from their chores to relax and nurse the baby.

A further obstacle to breastfeeding is their modest dress. Louisa proudly showed Elsie a nursing bra she'd made. It had 15 buttons down the front. Then there were the straightpins on her high-necked dress to deal with. Mennonites do not subscribe to zippers.

Sexuality and pregnancy are such private matters among the Mennonites, that a woman's sister would not necessarily know her due dates. Birth is not a family-centred event. Although the mother-in-law often lives in an extension of her son's farmhouse known as the "doddy house," she keeps a respectful distance at birthing time. Older children are whisked off to a neighbour if they are awake.

Peggy, the local buggymaker's wife, remembers how she and her husband Solomen had lots of questions to evade prior to their last home birth. Why were mommy and daddy moving the big bed into the kitchen alcove? "Because mommy might get sick," she'd laughed.

There was no discussion of birds or bees, so when four-year-old Stanley discovered infant Allen in bed the following morning he was astounded. "Is he ours? Where did he come from?" the child burst out. "Can we *keep* him?!"

Peggy tells the story with a broad smile stretched across her fine features. Then she illustrates her birthing history by pointing out heads among her lively brood of seven. "He was born at home. She was born at home. . .because *he* was born in the car."

The secret of birth is kept so long that one Old Order bishop confided in Violet's husband that he wished the midwives would teach the Mennonite young people. In a society that still practices "bundling," (under-the-covers dating with a barrier of blankets between the couple), the bishop's admission that people "don't always know how they get pregnant," takes on urgent significance.

Violet and Elsie are ready with information when it is called for. The younger midwife studies methods of natural birth control in anticipation of her clients' cautious enquiries. But the midwives must be subtle about this aspect of their work. After one woman haltingly asked how she might better space her family, a penitent note arrived in the midwife's mailbox. "Forgive me for having asked," the woman wrote. "I should never have thought of such a thing."

What women do learn about childbearing and rearing, is acquired during their service as "hired girls." A household with a new baby always takes on a neighbour's single daughter for six weeks of domestic help. These stints as hired girl provide a young woman with an apprenticeship in housewifery. Unfortunately, there is still no apprenticeship in midwifery.

Elsie and Violet reluctantly recognize that there should really be midwives among the Old Order women themselves. But up till now, no one has solved the dilemma of how a midwife could practice without a telephone. Perhaps one of those curious compromises with technology will soon be affected? Louisa has asked if she might "take some experience" with Elsie and Violet.

She, or another Old Order mother, will doubtless join the midwives' practice. It seems appropriate and inevitable. Meanwhile, Elsie and Violet, the women who brought birth back home for Mennonite babies, continue to bask in unparalleled appreciation. "Bless your work. . . ," "I thank you both heartily. . . ," "Wishing you courage to keep on. . . ," close the hand-scripted notes of thanks that keep arriving in their mailboxes. And from one elated farmer father, there is this message to other parents: "I wish God's Richest Blessing on all other people that want to try home birth."

Chapter Seven
Birth Stories and Midwives Musings

> Pregnant and birthing mothers are elemental forces, in the same
> way that gravity, thunderstorms, earthquakes and hurricanes are
> elemental forces. In order to understand the laws of their energy
> flow, you have to love and respect them for their magnificence, at
> the same time that you study them with the accuracy of a true scien-
> tist.
>
> — Ina May Gaskin

Matthieu, Marc, Luc and Benoit: One Mother's Birth Progression

My first childbirth experience was in October 1974. Everything went well during my pregnancy. I read a lot, went to prenatal classes and La Leche League meetings.

My waters ruptured around 5 p.m. and I got to hospital at 6 p.m. I had back pain and found that walking helped. At 8 p.m. I vomitted and then felt like having a bowel movement. They did a vaginal exam and found I was fully dilated. I had the urge to push, but they told me to wait.

Three doctors came in. A gynaecologist, a family doctor (not mine), and an intern. They did three rectal examinations, feeling the cord and the baby's feet. I went into the delivery room on my hands and knees without my husband. They did a pudendal block and the episiotomy. (I will never forget that feeling. I wasn't frozen.)

My first boy was born feet first, crying. They put him on my stomach, but since my hands were tied, I couldn't touch him.

I heard them say, "There's another one in here." By that time I had no urge to push and couldn't feel anything. They went for the forceps. I said I didn't want that and they explained they could not wait more than 20 minutes. I pushed hard. My second boy was born head first. Nineteen minutes between them. 5lb. 5 oz. and 4 lb. 11 oz. They kept them away from me for three days. I was able to see them through the window. I could also see the nurse giving them the bottle, even if I was pumping my milk every three hours for them. The head nurse told me I should relax.

On the fifth day we were home with Luc. They came to show me Matthieu. I had never held him. They said I could only look. My own child!

In January 1977 Marc was born. I decided on a doctor at the other hospital, since I heard they were more flexible. He agreed to no enema, no shave, nursing on the delivery table and rooming in. But I still had to have the episiotomy and stay at least three days.

Two days after my due date I felt pain in my back. We got to hospital, and when the nurse did a vaginal exam I felt my water rupture. She said I probably urinated; it was too early for my water to break. I had to go for a bowel movement. I told her it was time to call the doctor but she said there was no hurry.

I had an urge to push, so she checked me again and was surprised to find that I was fully dilated. She told me not to push (as if that was easy to do!). They brought me to the delivery room and put my feet in stirrups. This time they didn't tie my hands.

Emery was holding my hands, helping me to push, while I gave him a third son. The doctor came in just in time to do the episiotomy. He didn't cut as much, because I was able to sit down without pain within a week. (With the twins it took three weeks. And three months before we had sexual relations; I was so scared everything would tear again.)

When Marc was born I had no medication, the lights were down, and they let the baby nurse. They took him to the nursery for three hours, though I asked for him back sooner.

They wanted me to rest but I was so excited. I still nursed the twins; I couldn't wait to go home. The next morning I asked the doctor if I could go and he said it was impossible. So instead of being with my children I went to exercise class, nutrition class, and saw how to bath a baby!

They said two 2 1/2-year-old boys wouldn't notice that mother is away. I shouldn't worry about them! The next baby, I told myself, the children are coming with me.

Six years after, my dream came true. Home birth didn't appeal to me at first; I was scared something would happen. But after my best friend Anne-Marie had her fourth and fifth babies at home, I began to think positively about it.

I had changed doctors. I told him on my first visit that I was thinking of having the baby at home and he didn't see any problem. Only that I should have another Rhogam blood test done. I called a professor at the University of Moncton, and she sent me literature on it. I did take the Rhogam. My pregnancy went fine.

Our fourth boy was born at home with his family around him. It was so peaceful compared to the hospital. I woke up around 3 a.m. feeling some pressure on my cervix. Then the bloody show came out. The midwife told me to look for that and call then. I also called Anne-Marie. They came.

I had back pain so the midwife had me take to my hands and knees. She showed my husband how to rub my back. She was really calm and good to have around.

When I had an urge to push we woke up the children. My waters broke, and I stayed on my hands and knees for the delivery because that was comfortable; it was easier to push. Benoit's head was born. One last push and he was out.

Anne-Marie was holding my hands and my husband was talking to me and the children during the last minutes of the birth. I couldn't believe it was happening. We were so happy. I put Benoit to my breast.

It was the first time I was able to hold my baby so soon after birth. He was still warm and wet and he smelled so good. Emery cut the cord while the children watched attentively.

The midwife had to do a few stitches, since I tore a bit. One of my eight-year-old sons, noticing that it hurt while she was doing it, came and sat near me. He held my hand and patted my hair to make me feel better.

After that, Luc and Matthieu went to school, and Marc fell asleep with Benoit and I in our family bed.

Benoit is a contented baby. He is really calm; we noticed from the first day he was born.

Having no episiotomy didn't bother me at all. Two hours later I was sitting in a wooden chair having breakfast. What a difference!

— Andrée, Moncton, New Brunswick

Pregnancy and Personal Growth:

Pregnancy and birth have been a yardstick for me. Somehow they help me to evaluate my life. As we go through life we change. Some periods feel a bit stagnant, others are times of great growth. Because I've changed I react differently to each pregnancy. I open up more, become aware of myself.

It's like, here I am pregnant again. I was pregnant ten years ago, a very different person than I am now. Then I was pregnant two years later. I'd been through a lot of changes. Then six years and many changes later, pregnant once more. It's a measuring stick of my life.

— Dawn King

Unplanned Pregnancy:

Jim and I often talked about my feelings about the pregnancy and all. It took a few months, before I fully accepted it. While I no longer felt negative about it, neither did I feel positive. . . .I just accepted it and did what I had to do. I felt that I would never have the strong connection with this child that I did with Isaiah, whom I wanted from the very start, and who was not an unwelcome surprise. As with many things, it has been different than I expected. I feel very connected with her and love her deeply, much more than I ever thought I could.

— Dawn King

Elliot's Birth: A Family of Perspectives

I liked being with my Mom when she had the baby. It was exciting to watch the head come out. I felt really happy that I got a baby brother, and I was sure glad that everything went alright.

Thanks,
Jack, 10 years old

Everytime she pushed I got more excited. When he came out we all got our picture taken right away. We love him so much he hardly gets to go to sleep.

Sincerely,
Shane, 11 years old

I saw three babies be born and it got better all the time. Seeing Elliot be born made me appreciate him all the more. Instead of hearing all the exaggerated stories about birth, I saw first hand that it really isn't like that.

Thanks,
Steve, 13 years old

The morning of June 7th sticks out in my mind as one of my happiest. The birth of my son Elliot made me almost float with joy. Being able to hold my wife and really be involved with the birth (rubbing her back, holding hands and offering encouragement) made it a very touching experience. Watching my son emerge into this world brought tears to my eyes.

Sharing this experience with my sons brought us closer as a family in several ways. The bonding with our new son and the rest of the family was a truly beautiful occurance.

Our home birth brought a rare joy into our household, which I don't think will ever be equalled.

Robert

June 6th. I woke up with a backache. I didn't really think much of it until about an hour later when I had the slightest bit of blood-tinged discharge. My heart was doing cartwheels. I could hardly wait to call my midwife, but at the same time I was afraid to get my hopes up. As it was, nothing else really happened all that day. But Elsie did come and offered to stay the night just in case.

At 2:45 a.m. I felt a little pop and a tiny dribble of water escaped from my body. I went to the bathroom and a bit more gushed out. Soon the pains started and I awakened Elsie. She got up and calmly got things ready. We had a cup of tea and then she examined me. Things were happening fast. Violet was called, and also my sister, whom we had invited to the birth. The children were all sleeping.

I really don't remember much about the pain, but I will never forget the warm close feeling I had for everyone who was there. I felt like I was inside a bubble of love. I wasn't really aware of much.

At times I felt a little irritated and I had to remind myself that this was normal, "this was transition." Soon I felt an uncontrollable urge to push. The children were awakened. As soon as I saw them and heard their voices I got all tingly. I wanted this to be the most beautiful experience they could ever have.

With each push the crowd cheered. I felt like I was a gold medal winner in the Olympics. When the baby finally emerged, I thought I would be disappointed if I didn't have a girl, but I couldn't have been happier.

I nursed my little son and again I went into myself, but this time I took Bob and Elliot and my three big boys in with me. I felt wide open like a blanket. I wanted to wrap them all up together and hold them close to my heart. If I could live one day in my life over again, this is the day that I would choose.

Thanks so much Elsie and Violet.

Irene,
Kitchener-Waterloo, Ontario

Labour:

> Working in harmony with a client in labour is like making love. . .it's mirroring. . .you get in synch so you can anticipate their needs. Through that unity and symbiosis you evolve the comfort measures she needs.
>
> — Theo Dawson

> Labour is mysterious. The body knows and nobody else does. The key is to follow the woman.
>
> — Vicki van Wagner

Bonnie Johnson

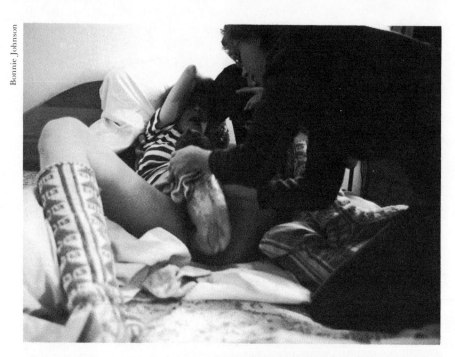

Midwife Bobbi catches Ben as Dale delivers.

Bonnie Johnson

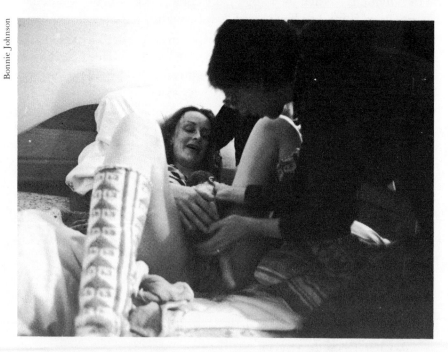

Dale greets her new son.

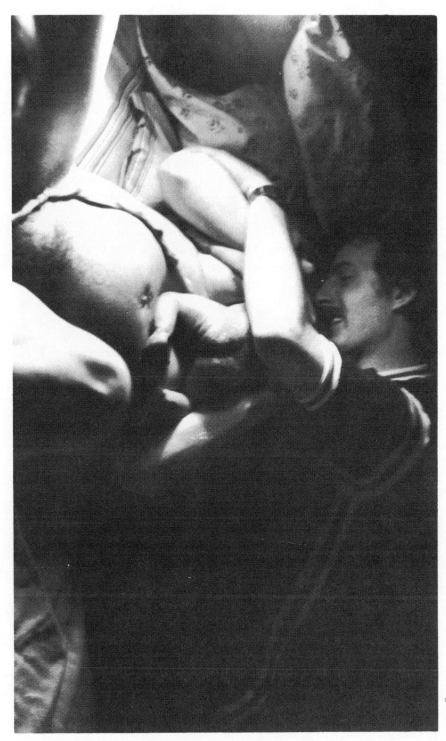

New father Martin enfolds his wife and infant.

Bonnie Johnson

Ryan's Home Birth

Sunday, November 9, 1980: Around 2 a.m. I got up a couple of times in a row to pee, half awake, wondering at my complete inability to control my bladder. The second time it hit me — my waters were leaking. First thought: I'm not ready for this. I felt panicky. Because I was in the bathroom such a long time, Eric called to me to see if I was O.K. I replied that I was leaking. Eric was half asleep, too, and it was a full minute before he realized I was referring to my waters and not my bladder. I came back to bed, asking for comfort, and we hugged for a little while. I started to relax, and then to get excited. The next time I went to the toilet I caught a glimpse of myself in the mirror, and I looked great. So this was it!

I lay in bed for a while with a towel between my legs, and soon started to feel very mild contractions. They were exactly like the Braxton-Hicks contractions I'd been having for the past few months. Sometime between 3:00 and 4:00 the contractions started coming every four or five minutes, and I started deep breathing through them. I realized that I wasn't going to be able to go back to sleep, so I got up, got dressed to keep warm, and went into the living room. I read, and day-dreamed, as the contractions gradually became stronger. At 6:00 I realized I was pretty tired, so I lay down on the couch and dozed until 6:45.

Until this time, although I knew I was in labour, I was reluctant to fully accept the fact. I think I was afraid of being disappointed if the whole thing turned out to be a sham. The acceptance came shortly after I awoke from my nap, partly because the contractions were fairly strong, and partly because I had set 7:00 as the time to call the midwives if things were proceeding.

I woke Eric up, then called Camille. My contractions increased in intensity and frequency through the morning, especially when I was walking around. I had to make eye contact with Eric to help me through them. By the time the midwives arrived around 12:30, I was glad to see them.

I continued walking around for a while, then lay down on the bed when walking got to be too much. Camille did an internal exam and said I was about three centimetres dilated. A while later Abra did one, and left her hand in during a contraction. She said she could feel the cervix open "beautifully" during the contraction.

The rest of the labour exists in my mind as a variety of impressions, without a definite sequence. Lying on the bed with an abundance of pillows, Eric holding my left hand and Paulina my right, breathing through contractions looking into Abra's eyes. Eric softly reminding me to relax my arms, my neck, my forehead. Camille saying to let the contractions go through me, and me repeating "through me" during the next contraction. Thinking, and saying, "open" in a drawn-out breath while my mind focussed on my cervix. The loss of control when I had to throw up in the middle of a very long contraction. The beautiful, positive feelings in the room, focussed on me and my baby. Eric rubbing my buttocks where the muscle was really tight. Abra saying, "There's just a rim left from 12:30 to 8:00 o'clock."

Then second stage: me following the lead from my uterus, my entire body responding to the force within. Abra saying, "You have a beautiful body for birthing." Camille whispering suggestions in my ear: "Send oxygen to the baby," "Keep your voice low," and me integrating her words into the experience.

Changing positions: squatting on the floor through one contraction, and feeling the baby's head drop right down; on all fours for a couple of contractions, but that didn't feel right, so back onto my back. The burning sensation in my perineum as the baby's head showed more and more. George holding the mirror so I could see what was happening. Abra suggesting I put my hand on the baby's head as it was coming out (warm and wet). His head crowning, and then being outside me.

It wasn't until the head was born, and George moved with the mirror so I could see the face, that I really believed I was going to have a baby. I felt an incredible rush of joy. I said, "Look, Eric, he's really here," and I think I cried. Abra delivered the anterior shoulder, then the rest of the upper body. She asked me if I wanted to catch him, and I put my hands down. One more push, then he was out and onto my chest. A blanket over us, him crying a little, me massaging the vernix into his back and limbs. Eric and I looking into his eyes, open wide in the darkness. Ryan had arrived.

— Karen,
Nelson, B.C.

Labour Pain:

> Often people who are into painless childbirth cite the example of native ladies who are out working in the fields, squat, give birth to their baby, and then go back to work. The assumption is that they have no pain, that it is easy for them, and that it could be that way for us. I have always accepted that theory. Now, after some thought, it seems to me that maybe what is happening with that lady is not that she isn't experiencing pain but that her attitude towards pain is different than ours. She accepts it and doesn't complain about it, doesn't get into feeling sorry for herself. I did that too, but

the pain was there and certainly very real. I don't see how it could be otherwise.

The doctor whose relaxation class we went to said, "The uterus only produces pressure, not pain." I filed that one away in my head for awhile. Then I thought, pressure can definitely produce pain. If you have 100 lbs. of pressure on your foot, no matter how relaxed you are, how unafraid you are, how much you've practised your deep breathing, it's likely going to hurt.

— Dawn King

Alison: A Triumphant VBAC

In 1975, I gave birth to our first child, Jason, by cesarean. In 1977, our daughter, Sondra, was born also by cesarean section.

Five years later I found myself pregnant again. I inquired into the possibility of having a trial of labour and was counselled by several people to go the route of the obvious: once a section, always a section. In approaching the GP whom I was seeing at the time, I was told not once, but twice, that I, as well as the child, might die. An obstetrician in Prince George told me that I had a "funnel pelvis." He reluctantly agreed to a trial of labour but strongly advised another section.

We then got a referral to a doctor in Vancouver who was recommended to us. He (bless him!) told me that my body was normal, and he didn't see why I couldn't try it, although there was some hesitation because of the two previous sections.

Two weeks before my due date, we headed to Vancouver (500 miles away). The week passed with nary a twinge! My due date came and went. After another week and a half, my doctor was beginning to be concerned, so he ordered daily fetal heart strips. That didn't help my morale any, especially when the heart rate dipped below 120 a couple of times.

On a Friday afternoon, I began having contractions fifteen minutes apart. By midnight Saturday, I was sure this was it. This time I had continued "business as usual," eating and resting so my strength was there when I needed it. By 6:30 a.m. we phoned Laurie, who in turn phoned the midwife. When the midwife arrived, I was 7 cm.

The next few hours seemed to pass very slowly, and I began to wonder why I had not opted for the section. But Laurie and my midwife were very supportive, encouraging me with each contraction, and helping me to find the most comfortable position. Somewhere around 9 cm they thought that if I would squat, my waters would break and dilation would speed up. They did break, and I felt it would not be too much longer.

We had decided (Ken and I) beforehand that we would wait as long as possible to go into the hospital, as we preferred the relaxed atmosphere of the home in which we were staying. As well, we wanted as little interference as possible, and our doctor wasn't on call that weekend. After all, I had been down there a month. With all the expense involved and the separation from the children, we didn't want to end up with a section.

At 11:30 the midwife announced all systems "go," and I could push. After all that time, it felt good; I was on the home stretch! So with a housecoat on, I was assisted to the car by my husband. The midwife followed in her own car. We were only twelve minutes from Grace Hospital and traffic was light, so the trip to the hospital went without a hitch.

Upon arriving, they hustled me into the birthing chair. The resident was called, and I could push to my heart's content. After some time, the nurse reported the heart rate dropping to 90, so they advised us that it would be best to get the baby out as soon as possible. We agreed to an episiotomy. One half hour after arrival at the hospital, Alison was born. We did it.

Ken held her while they stitched me up, and the bonding began. The next day, we asked for an early discharge since I felt so good. Monday afternoon we were on our way home.

I felt good, and by Friday my stitches were healed up. What a contrast to my previous cesarean! No one can convince me, as they tried to do before, that a cesarean is easier than labour. Sure, labour is hard work, and painful as well, but the results — the shorter healing period, my feelings toward myself, my husband and baby — were well worth the extra effort!!

— Lila,
Vanderhoof, B.C.

Death at Birth:

> I was terrified of death. My head was filled with horrid images. I did not know that there is a quiet, peaceful beauty in death. That the colours of death are not vile, but different. That death is bitterly sad but survivable. I reached out and touched that first stillborn babe and the spell of fear and ugliness was broken. My heart opened. My desire to run away was replaced by a flood of tears.
>
> — Theo Dawson

Kevin's Story: Postpartum Concerns

We decided to have our second child at home. As the months went by I became increasingly frustrated at the medical system that had put us in a position of having to be deceitful about where the child was to be born and the name of the doctor who was taking care of me.

When I saw our local doctor he told me he didn't approve of home birth as he didn't feel safe in the home environment and so would not do prenatal checks. I said I didn't feel safe in the hospital. When I had routine blood tests done I had to name a hospital in order to cause no problems for the midwife involved or ourselves. In order to get medical back-up we needed referrals from one doctor to another and I got the distinct impression that fees were the relevant point and not our welfare. We could find very little help from the medical profession in having a baby at home but at the eleventh hour our local doctor said he would come out if necessary. He realized I was determined to have a home birth if possible and as he said, he didn't want any heroes.

We were pleased at his offer and hoped to have him as an ally to home birth in the future. It was necessary to call him out for some assistance with suturing, and he came promptly to the home at 11 p.m.

We took our son for a check-up to the same doctor three days later and he was concerned about jaundice. When we told him the icterometer had indicated a bilirubin level of 10, he said that it was high and should be checked again and went on to explain that if the level was any higher he would have to be hospitalized, put under bili lights and fed only glucose water. We were to go straight to the hospital from his office.

He further explained that he would be brain damaged as a result of not getting the bilirubin level down but it could be avoided if we acted immediately. While we were at the hospital, he wanted him x-rayed to check a possible displaced hip. He said he would be crippled for life and we should double diaper him for six months and then have him x-rayed again.

We were very concerned with what he had told us but decided to go home and discuss things first. We consulted midwives and other doctors and decided to get the bilirubin level checked again and then make a decision about getting treatment in hospital. The doctor was waiting for us when we got to the hospital an hour later and we got VIP treatment because of the urgency of the case. We had declined to have Kevin x-rayed and had decided to consult a pediatrician instead. Two hours later the doctor called us at home to say the count was 14 and he had made arrangements for Kevin to go under the lights and for me to stay with him as I was breastfeeding.

We explained that we wanted to treat him at home and allow his body to eliminate the jaundice as nature had intended, and that I would nurse him on demand to help him do this. The doctor was appalled. He said that he would take no responsibility for our brain damaged child and that we had no right to disregard his advice. It took three to four years to recognize signs of further complications if he got worse and it would be too late by the time we acted.

He wanted to know who had been advising us and when we said we had consulted with our midwife he said she was practising medicine illegally. We told him that another doctor's opinion had been considered when we made our decision and this made him angry. He finally told us he would put in writing that he wanted nothing more to do with us and our brain damaged baby and he hung up.

He would not even sign the inevitable piece of paper that would allow us to take Kevin to the local hospital the next day to confirm that the bilirubin level was being reduced by the natural process. So we had to deal with a more understanding doctor and go to another hospital 40 minutes away. We did put Kevin under lights for a few hours at home and I nursed him frequently. The next test showed the level down from 14, the highest it ever reached, to 12.5 and this confirmed that his system was dealing with it as intended, with little intervention.

At no time did our midwife or her assistant tell us what to do. They calmly answered our questions and supplied the information necessary to make our own decision. They told us they would support us no matter what we decided, i.e., hospital or home care.

The doctor had reported us to the health authorities and a public health nurse phoned us on the sixth day to say she wanted to visit in half an hour. I explained it was not convenient and after trying to insist, she agreed to call the following day. She confirmed that Kevin was dealing with the jaundice and that we were caring parents who had acted responsibly in the best interest of our baby. She said she would visit us next week but we didn't hear from her again. She was obviously not concerned with brain damage or the way we were dealing with the situation.

If we were not informed and did not have the support and care of our midwife/friends, we might have gone along with the doctor and hospitalized a baby that did not need it, put him in an incubator, given him glucose water, interfered with the initial important stages of breastfeeding, had him x-rayed at three days old, not to mention being separated from my two-year-old at an important time. I can only assume that the doctor had the baby's best interest at heart, but that being the case, he should become more educated about jaundice, the importance of nursing and the family unit.

We had a slight insight into the heartbreak and distress that can be caused when a doctor gives people bad news. We had no problem at all, but he almost had us believing our baby was brain damaged. He used the term frequently, and said that Kevin could be a cripple for life because of a possible displaced hip which was found to be normal by a pediatrician.

My heart goes out to those parents who do have a problem and I hope they find understanding medical and family support. I would like to take this opportunity to express our thanks and appreciation to the midwives for their care and help at a time when it was most needed.

— Evelyn,
Aldergrove, B.C.

Time At Birth:

> During a birth time disappears. It's a strange thing. Like when you're making love or drunk.
>
> — June Chenard

Birth and Spirituality:

> At a birth you feel a divine energy flow right through all of you. It's like an electrical buzz. . .the energy of life flowing into the baby.
>
> — Abra Palumbo

Sean: Home Labour to Hospital Birth

7:00 a.m. A sunny Saturday. The figure of a round woman clad only in a large t-shirt and heavy woolen socks stands in the middle of a kitchen, hugged by three people. Memory: I am not alone. We will do this together.

10:00 a.m. The woman sits cross-legged while sun hits the carpet below her. Two sets of hands rest on her knees. Hands of midwives. The room resonates with the ebb and flow of their sighs. Memory: It is a circle of caring. I feel my baby coming.

10:45 a.m. A man, two women and a cat sprawl on a king sized bed focussing on the moans coming from the head beneath the pillow. Memory: Light strokes tenderly soothing down my legs.

11:15 a.m. The back seat of a taxi filled with round woman, her man and midwife while the front seat holds driver and midwife. Destination: the hospital. Mission accomplished via the mania of College Street on a sunny, shopping, Saturday afternoon. Memory: the eyes of John and the reassuring touch of the back-seat midwife.

12:00 noon. The round woman sits upright on a hospital bed with an arm around the necks of her partner and a midwife. She pushes life through herself and almost out of the people beside her as they support her. Another midwife stands in front flowing with each change. Memory:

My body is not my own. Rhythmically, I give myself up to this power. I need the gentle continuum of her care and the strength of my partner.

1:37 p.m. The round woman presses into the bed. He is here. It's over. The midwife softly urges her to reach for the quiet, little human between her legs. Heads touching, midwife and mother, suckling child. Memory: Large round eyes staring up at me as he travels to my breast. We massage his slippery skin. Timeless. Thank-you, Chris. Thank-you, Patty.

— Holly,
Toronto, Ontario

Birth and Sexuality:

> The one thing you can compare with giving birth, is making love. There are a hundred ways to compare them. We midwives accept the sexual aspects of birth.
>
> — Isabelle Brabant

Intuition:

> Intuition is the totality of everything I have ever seen, experienced, learned and felt.
>
> — Theo Dawson

Mark's Birth: Prepared Cesarean

My first child was born at the Mount Sinai Hospital in December 1977. I was so badly treated by the obstetrician only the dream of a home birth gave me the courage to conceive again.

I should explain that I am from British Guyana, South America. We used the British midwifery system. My mother had ten children at home. My mother's mother also had ten children at home.

I got together with midwife Theo Dawson, anticipating a home birth. However, one week before delivery, the baby became a footling breech. After twelve hours of labour, an emergency cesarean section was performed.

I praise the Lord for a beautiful healthy baby and for a midwife who gave me something called empathy.

Theo prepared me psychologically for the cesarean experience. She advised me to choose certain options. She also allowed me to take my five-year-old son to the hospital where she babysat him while I was undergoing hospital procedures. My elder son was able to see the baby half an hour after birth.

Theo's presence was a comfort to my husband. He was able to relax and concentrate on our two children, knowing that I was in the care of the midwife.

Lastly, it was Theo who insisted that I nurse the baby as soon as I was taken from the recovery room to the hospital room. She knew that mother/infant bonding had not taken place because of the anaesthetic and the surgery. I was tired and disinterested in the baby. She made sure that I nursed the baby before she left the hospital. It was the breastfeeding which helped my feelings to return. The more I nursed, the better I felt. I would advise every birthing woman to have a midwife, inside or outside the hospital.

I enjoyed being pampered and comforted by my midwife.

May God's wrath fall on all those who oppose the legalization of midwifery.

— Rrana,
Scarborough, Ontario

Home Birth Babies:

> When I catch a baby I have a feeling that there's a whole new breed being born. . . .gentle, self-determined, hearts of gold. These kids are here on the planet right now to do some real saving work.
> — Judi Pustil

Birth and Universality:

> Birth is like an echo. Each baby is my child. Is me. Is my own mother giving birth to me. Each mother is myself giving birth. Her fears and her opening heart are mine too. We are all simultaneously experiencing it.
> — Abra Palumbo

Liam's Birth: Home Plans and Hospital Transfer

Saturday, about 11:30 p.m.: I got up from bed and accepted that labour was starting with good strong back contractions. My partner helped me deal with them and about 1:30 a.m. went out to get the midwife. My time alone felt fine. The breathing was successful; I felt positive and confident. When partner and midwife arrived, I was in bed. All was quiet with the air full of the birth spirit.

At 2 a.m. I went to the bathroom where the waters broke in three clear gushes. I dealt with the contractions more calmly and they didn't seem to reach the intensity of my first labour. I vomitted a few times and knew the obvious signs of transition were present.

Early Sunday morning: Midwife found 4-5 cm dilation and that the baby was moving from the right backside to the front so we could see a lumpish rise above the public bone. Midwife called for a back-up team of nurse and a coach, who arrived smiling and encouraging. It felt good to have fresh energy and positive vibrations.

At noon I was moving around a great deal, and walking felt good. Lots of physical contact and support from the coaching team. Back massage helped ease the muscle tension. The baby's head was seen passing the sacrum as a small soft ball. I was able to pee often and found the physical support of the coaching team encouraged me.

At 2:45 p.m. partner and I were together a while. I took some juice and had a bowel movement, which lightened the pressure. My older son was around with one other youngster and I found I welcomed the kids. By late afternoon I was beginning to tire and felt the urgency to get it on. Midwife and coach team were concerned by the delayed second stage and wondered what the block was. Another internal and full dilation was here with no cervix. But midwife felt a soft bulge which could be an anterior lip. Oddball presentation, i.e., brow ear, etc., comes to mind and stayed with midwife. Meanwhile I had no urge to push. There was a mound of pillows on the bed to lean on while on my hands and knees. My pulse was high at 120 so an electro drink, labourade, was given. It tasted great and brought my pulse to 100. The contractions were varied, but with eye contact of the coaching team I managed.

By early evening there were still no urges to push and we phoned the Lasqueti Island midwife and talked awhile. She urged change. Sitting outside, where there is more oxygen, for an hour, gave a change of energy. I felt frustrated because of no progress. After a reminder to collect my psychic energy and use my power to push my baby out, I decided to get help.

There was a sad feeling, but I was too tired and no end was near. Drove to Comox with midwife in back helping me cope with contractions. The maternity ward was quiet. About ten minutes were spent in a small room until a nurse confirmed the midwife's findings of full dilation. With good heartbeat and blood pressure we were wheeled into delivery.

Then I understood the green and gold sensations I had had all through the pregnancy. The delivery room walls, gowns, linens etc. were green and gold. This and having my partner and midwife with me in gowns helped ease the tensions, and I felt comfortable. The doctor came and our team of five occupied the O.R. for five hours waiting for the baby to emerge. I pushed mightily with contractions every ten minutes, with three good pushes to each.

A change to hands and knees, still breathing comfortably, maintained the energy. Doctor's hands were in and out of my vagina. Wishfully thinking the baby's head would flex and descend. An ear was presenting and the head was transverse. After 3 1/2 hours, forceps seemed close. Dr. B. called the obstetrician who arrived at 1:05 a.m.

After five hours of pushing, different position, two tables, I ended up on the delivery table with a wedge at my back to prop me up. Making some sounds helped me to release air and energy but the nurse wanted me to maintain efficiency and hold my breath while pushing. This felt strained but she was forceful and things went her way.

The obstetrician arrived and efficiently took over with an unhurried operation set up. The wedge was removed and I laid with my feet in stirrups, with my partner and midwife at my head for eye contact and support. The energy was calm and good and I was relaxed as can be. After the anesthetic I felt most of the freezing was on the outside with gradually less freezing up inside. The midwife gave a valuable connection, keeping me centred on the baby while still feeling my own body. The birth remained mine. With the cuts to the rear, in two contractions the forceps were in. They turned the head. It crowned with the next contraction and came up with lots of dark hair.

My partner and midwife saw a flat large beautiful face with vernix and pale bluish colour. The pushing was so different from my first baby. It felt very dry coming down the canal and hurt so I yelled and cried with joy. The baby was born with the next contraction while I trembled, whimpered, releasing and reaching. "Give me my baby," and I held him for imprinting. There was no orgasmic release as with my first birth. The body of the mother came back to itself and the body of the baby was free. Thanks to the great spirit.

My partner gently rubbed and caressed, shielding and talking to the boy who was all quiet and wrapped up. This is a bond to replace not catching the baby, as he did our first. Everyone is surprised at the baby's size (10 lbs. 9 1/2 oz).

Afterwards we had a private room so we could all remain together and talk of the birth. The baby sucked lustily at my breast. After a rest we left for home later that morning.

— Pat,
Vancouver Island, B.C.

Midwife's Dreams:

> I dreamt about one birth, a forceps delivery in hospital, for two
> weeks. I dream births over and over. They stop at the same place or
> get a little farther, 'til they're resolved.
>
> — Jane Cocks

A Protective Aura:

> One of the most powerful ways to help a couple who are apprehen-
> sive about the hospital is to encourage a vision of how loved and pro-
> tected she can feel. I tell her it will be as if there is an aura of love and
> trust and protective strength surrounding her. When we move from
> their home to the hospital, we move within that aura. At the
> hospital, she continues to labour within it, inviting hospital person-
> nel to enter her space periodically when necessary. With this vision
> she pictures an environment in which she can feel safe.
>
> — Bobbi Soderstrom

Matthieu: In Hospital and In Control

I had a fantastic hospital birth, largely due to my midwife. On a warm
July day my husband, mother and midwife were all sharing labour with
me in our little home. All was going well and smoothly when suddenly,
things started moving fast and already I could feel the baby's head in the
birth canal.

The drive to the hospital was enjoyable, much to my surprise. The
hard contractions stopped and the night air blew gently on my face. I
held the midwife's hand while my husband drove and my mother looked
on. I'll never forget what the midwife said: "All four of us have created
an atmosphere, a sort of aura, and we must keep it alive. We will open up
a little and include the doctor (whom I like very much) in our aura.
Nothing else will penetrate it."

When we got to the hospital my husband dropped us off at the door but
we waited for him as he parked the car so our aura wouldn't get broken
up. Up we went all together. I felt so protected. I didn't have to interact
with anyone; everything was so well taken care of. And there was the
doctor waiting with a glowing smile on his face; he was already part of
our aura. Twenty minutes later our son was born in a dimly lit room.
Our glowing aura was gentle enough to his eyes. An hour later, as arranged, we were home again. Our son is so beautiful, fresh, peaceful —
and glowing.

Thank you, Bobbi.

— Margo,
Ottawa, Ontario

A Midwife's Role:

> Spread love
> The saving grace
> On the wounded
> Weeping World.
> Weeping, washing tears,
> Cleansing, repenting,
> Replenishing.
>
> — Sandra Botting

"Alison," "Kevin" and "Liam" first printed in *Maternal Health News*. "Sean" first printed in *Issue*. Reproduced here with permission of the publications.

Chapter Eight
Safety, Risk and Medical Opinion

Absolute safety in birth is not to be found anywhere. There is always a trade-off of risks. . . . Safety has become such an overriding consideration for the medical profession that it passes the point of no return, and perhaps we cause more hazards than we correct.

— *Dr. Murray Enkin,*
Professor of Obstetrics & Gynaecology,
McMaster University

B irth is a major life transformation, and like any change of such magnitude, it involves elements of uncertainty and risk. No country, no maternity care system and no practitioner can claim to eliminate the risks of childbirth. While, reassuringly, 85-90% of all normal pregnancies will resolve themselves without complications and without interventions in healthy births, a small percentage of infants do require assistance to survive and thrive, and a tragic few mothers and babies are still lost each year. That tiny tragic minority makes physical safety the focus of concern about all childbirth practices.

The amplified voice of popular wisdom in our society declares that only medically-attended hospital births, with up-to-date obstetrical technology on hand, can be truly safe. Lately a vociferous whisper of public dissent is giving evidence that other childbirth options might indeed be as safe or safer.

Part of this difference of opinion is due to the varying interpretations of the word "safety." Some would reduce it to a simple matter of mortality: a life or death definition. The medical profession usually evaluates safety with mortality and morbidity statistics. (The latter measure birth injuries and illnesses that do not cause death.)

Many parents, doctors and health professionals now evaluate safety in a much wider context. Included in the equation are long-term physical, psychological and developmental consequences of the perinatal period. Some of these are caused by risks inherent in childbirth, others by the medical interventions which impose new risks on normal childbirth. Doris Haire, former President of the International Childbirth Education Association, applies the long-term parameters of safety when she says, "If you want to know what has gone wrong in obstetrics, read the pediatric journals."[1]

The medical profession has done a laudable job of reducing maternal and infant mortality in recent years. Canada has climbed to a respectable eighth on the World Health Organization's Infant Mortality Rate scale (considered to be the best cross-cultural indicator of birth out-comes). However, in conscientiously striving to eliminate the death risk in childbirth, the medical system has inadvertently introduced new safe-ty risks. Ever in search of improved infant mortality statistics, medicine has developed myopia about long-term safety indicators, and blindness to important psychological, developmental and social consequences of pregnancy and birth.

Brilliant medical technology developed to protect a few high risk mothers and babies is increasingly applied to the normal birthing popu-lation on a just-in-case rationale. Unfortunately each technical, chemical or surgical intervention carries its own risks. That risk may be entirely justified in a life-saving context, but is at best questionable as a supposedly preventative measure. Indeed, various high risk obstetrical interventions are now being proven unsafe for the low risk mother and child.

Given the current norms of obstetrical intervention, the conscientious parent approaching childbirth has such extra safety factors to assess as: fetal depression due to drugs received during labour; increased chances of maternal infection and mortality due to the high cesarean rate (18.5% in Ontario in 1983); and a greater possibility of brain damage due to routine use of obstetrical forceps. Dr. Caldero Barcia, former head of the International Confederation of Gynaecology & Obstetrics, goes so far as to state that "iatrogenia [doctor-caused illness] is the main cause of fetal distress."[2]

The medical definition of safety rarely includes psychological factors, though it is increasingly difficult to separate the psychological effects of birth from their developmental consequences. In his paper "Birth: Im-pact on the Participants," psychiatrist Dr. David Mandel asks if physical safeguards to mother and infant can be more important than their emotional growth and well being. As a society, shouldn't we expect both?

He points out animal and human studies on parent-child bonding as examples. Goats and sheep, separated from their offspring at birth, will not accept them later. Mothers separated from their infants at birth ap-parently do not receive some important cues to maternal behaviour, and thus a lack of bonding time is associated with child abuse, neglect and non-organic failure-to-thrive. In contrast, the five-year-old children of "extra early contact" mothers have higher I.Q.'s and advanced results on language tests. Other studies suggest that mothers who receive solicitous care during labour are less likely to reject their babies, and that the mother's birthing experience is related to the infant's motor and cognitive development at two and six months. Good feelings about a birth would appear to enhance her mothering capacities, and therefore her child's development.

The social consequences of birth practices reach into many dark corners of Canadian life. Surely any valid assessment of safety must include the child's physical safety from parental abuse. A serious analysis of the long-term effects of obstetrics asserts that: "Studies of battered babies suggest that some aspects of obstetrical management may have such grave consequences that they must be considered as seriously as factors which are known to cause perinatal death."[3]

The child whose parent lacks emotional support, who is deprived of bonding time or born prematurely, is more susceptable to anti-social behaviour later in life. The violence inflicted on an infant, be it physical or psychological, is often visited back on society by a disturbed adult. A 1980 Senate Royal Commission investigating the causes of criminal behaviour devoted a whole book, *Child At Risk*, to perinatal and early childhood factors.

Thus it is difficult to dismiss parents' concern about their own and their baby's experience of birth as strictly secondary to the medical definition of safety. The risks of any chosen birth attendant or place of birth must be weighed against the available alternatives. Within these scales, the current consumer definition of safety might include the inherent risks of the birth process to physical safety and survival, iatrogenic risks, and psycho-social risks. Parents weigh each factor according to their own consciences and priorities.

Given the complexity of the whole risk question, it is no wonder that most parents still abdicate their choices to the medical experts, as society advises. Medicalized, hospitalized birth may not always be the "safest" choice (given a broad definition to the term), but it is certainly the route of least resistance.

Nevertheless, more and more parents are making birthing choices a priority, because they realize that they must live with the long-term responsibility for consequences. They judge alternative caregivers against the backdrop of current medical weaknesses and strengths. They recognize that medical progress on the mortality front has afforded us the luxury of seeking an overall better birth experience, and a holistic definition of safety. While acknowledging a large debt to medical accomplishment, they refuse to be held hostage to the past. In the name of evolution, they demand for themselves and their children the best possible birth.

The International Reputation of Midwifery

World Health Organization statistics demonstrate that those industrialized countries with the most extensive midwifery services have the best birth outcomes, regardless of the place of birth. Sweden, consistently ranking best on the Infant Mortality Rate (IMR) scale (1981: 7 per 1,000), employs midwives for all pregnant women, even those high risk cases who will eventually be delivered by an obstetrician. In the Netherlands, where most women have midwives, 38% do not even see a doctor, and more than a third of births occur at home. The IMR in 1981 was an impressive 8.2 per 1,000. The cesarean section rate was notably only one quarter of the Canadian rate (less than 5% compared to almost 20%). Canada's IMR that year was 9.6 per 1,000, and the U.S., with its aggressive obstetrical trends, rated an embarrassing 11.7 per 1,000.[4]

Many studies have demonstrated the superior outcomes of midwifery care. Childbirth alternatives advocate David Stewart cites evidence from several European countries and thirteen American states in his book *The Five Standards of Safe Childbearing*. One of the most revealing studies compares birth statistics of general practitioners, (G.P.s), nurse-midwives (N.M.s) and obstetricians (O.B.s) working with the same high risk population in Madera County, California over subsequent time periods.

	1959 G.P.s	1960-63 N.M.s	1964-66 O.B.s
Neonatal Mortality Rate (per 1,000 live births)	23.9	10.3	32.1
Prematurity Rate (percentage)	11.0	6.4	9.8

The birthing population was served by general practitioners until 1960, when a nurse-midwifery program was instituted. It, in turn, was cancelled in 1963 at the behest of the medical association, in spite of its impressive results. The obstetricians who took over fared very badly. Only dangerous interventive obstetrics and a real lack of preventative prenatal care could explain such an appalling deterioration in the statistics.[5]

The lay midwives of "The Farm" spiritual community in Tennessee have demonstrated the safety of their practice over ten years and 1,200 low and high risk births. The prematurity rate among this well-cared-for maternity population was only 3%, and neonatal complications affected only 2.3% of the babies. Their cesarean section rate was 1.8%, only 5 babies out of 1,200 were delivered with forceps, and 95% of the women were able to deliver at home or in The Farm clinic. Farm statistics consistently bettered the perinatal mortality statistics for their state.[6]

Dr. Lewis Mehl studied a matched population of 421 women attended by lay midwives at home with 421 women attended by physicians in hospital, concluding that low risk mothers were better off at home with non-interventionist midwives: "The midwife sample had significantly less fetal distress, meconium staining, post-partum hemorrhage, birth injuries and infants requiring resuscitation. . .also higher mean APGAR scores." (Rating for baby's state of health at one and five minutes after birth.) A subsequent part of the study compared the physician-attended population for interventionist techniques, and postulates that lower rates of intervention resulted in better birth outcomes.[7]

Another Mehl study, the best existing controlled scientific evaluation of the safety of home versus hospital birth, compared 1,046 low risk women planning hospital births attended by general practitioners or obstetricians, and those having home births with lay midwives, nurse-midwives or general practitioners. Home and hospital populations fared equally on mortality scales, but morbidities were startlingly lower among the home birth population, particularly those attended by lay midwives.[8] This study is not conclusive scientific proof that home birth is safer for low risk populations, but it does once again point out the effectiveness of nature-trusting midwifery care.

Whether nurse-midwives or lay, attending at home or in hospital, the weight of evidence indicates that midwifery care promises the best birth outcomes among low — and some high — risk populations. Because of the non-status of midwifery in Canada, no study has yet determined that our midwifery care is equally superior. No group of midwives has yet compiled a birth count large enough to be statistically significant. But both the anecdotal evidence and what statistics do exist point to results similar to the U.S. experience.

Two Edmonton nurse-midwives who have attended several hundred home births report these statistics for 245 births: 87% of the women were able to complete their home deliveries as planned; there were no maternal or infant deaths among the home or hospital births; the group resulted in a cesarean section rate of 4.4% and a forceps rate of only 2.4%; APGAR scores for the babies averaged 8.1 out of 10 at one minute, and 9.6 out of 10 at five minutes.[9]

In the entire history of the new midwifery in Canada, after a dozen years and many thousands of births, there have been no known instances of maternal mortality. Perinatal mortalities, including those caused by congenital abnormalities have been surprisingly rare, even in the early days of inexperienced midwifery. Since any infant death subsequent to a home birth attracts immediate media attention, and usually legal investigation too, it is unlikely that fatal midwifery outcomes would have escaped the public eye, or the critical examination of medical bodies.

The first pilot study of midwifery care in Canada, conducted at the Grace Hospital in Vancouver in 1983-84, has shown encouraging results thus far. The midwives working with obstetrical supervision have halved intervention rates of obstetrical services in the province, and boast a far higher incidence of natural, vaginal births.[10] To say nothing of the reportedly high level of consumer satisfaction.

Why Midwifery is Safer

Midwifery care is not "safe" in any absolute sense. Midwives err like any other practitioners and some situations are beyond their scope of expertise. But at present, several factors make their style of care less risky for most mothers than modern obstetrics, even taking into account the exchange of risks involved in home births.

First, the home birth population is carefully screened by midwives for any high risk potential. Since the majority of midwife births are still happening at home, this screening process improves potential outcomes. It is an essential safety factor in home birth. Midwives work with higher risk clients in hospital only.

Prenatal care is crucial in keeping the low risk pregnancy in that category, and reducing the odds against a high risk mother. In a five- to ten-minute visit, it is virtually impossible for an obstetrician to question, assess and direct a mother's diet, exercise, psychological state, family situation, and all the other indicators of potential pregnancy and birth complications.

Nor can he really develop the compassionate and trusting relationship conducive to effective birth support. Some family doctors are able to more closely approximate midwifery prenatal care, monitoring more than mere vital signs, but the nature of the medical timetable works against them. Rarely do physicians have the nutritional knowledge most midwives cultivate, and nutrition during pregnancy is increasingly recognized as the single most important factor in determining birth outcomes.[11]

Midwives are able to work more directly with the psychological variables that affect a woman's bodily process in labour. Because of her preferred position as friend and confidante, the midwife is able to help her clients work through mental blocks that can interfere with labour. Unresolved feelings about an old abortion, fear of the responsibilities of motherhood, or inhibitions about her exposed state are among the reasons why a labour "fails to progress," thus threatening the baby's well-being. A midwife can apply astute questions where a doctor would apply forceps. She can also create a warm environment in which her client relaxes, is less tense, and thus experiences less pain and resistance to the flow of labour. The presence of a lay woman has been demonstrated to improve birth outcomes.[12]

Continuity of care is another major safety factor that medical practitioners rarely approximate. The time and frequency of contact between midwife, mother-to-be, and her family allow the midwife to develop an understanding of the physical and psychological norms of the individual client. This familiarity leads to early detection of deviations from those norms. Often a minor action or direction can correct an off-track labour at this point. Without a vigilant midwife, it might be allowed to develop into a full-scale complication before it is noted by the overworked ward nurse. The doctor, who hopefully knows his patient too, may not even be in the hospital at the time.

Midwives are trained to appreciate nature's ability to correct many problems during labour. Patterns of contractions or progress that appear odd at any point do not immediately necessitate a medical take-over. The woman herself may somehow adjust the aberration. The midwife watches and judges whether intervention is appropriate. Often the problem disappears. Doctors may be mystified, but the midwife is not surprised. Lay Midwife and Masters of Nursing student Jennifer Stonier has observed that, ''In the medical model, the healthy resolution of complications is understood as spontaneous remission or chance. Really, nature and the woman are coping and correcting, intentionally and naturally.

But as Lewis Mehl's study indicated, perhaps the most important factor in making midwifery relatively safer than medicine, for normal and low risk women, is avoidance of popular medical interventions. The American Academy of Pediatrics Committee on Drugs has declared that ''no drug has been proven safe for the unborn child,''[13] yet the overwhelming majority of women still receive anaesthetics, analgesics or hormone drugs in the course of hospital labours. The U.S. FDA has pointed out that the effects of ultrasound at the cellular level are significant enough that, were it a drug or substance, it would be labelled carcinogenic. A study on the bioeffects of ultrasound advises that ''we need more information on both safety and efficacy before we can endorse the unrestrained use of ultrasound during pregnancy.[14] Yet women with normal pregnancies are now routinely being invited to ''have a look at their babies'' once, twice, even three times during their terms.

Rupture of the membranes is one common medical practice to speed up labour. Dr. Caldero-Barcia looks at the time saved and the associated morbidities and asks: ''Is it worthwhile to reduce labour by 30-40 minutes at the expense of all the deformation and possible damage to the head of the fetus?''[15]

Electronic fetal heart monitors are routinely attached to mothers in labour, although they restrict her movement and comfort. The monitors frequently slip or malfunction, and they are often used to reduce the necessary time and attention of an obstetrical nurse. They provide no more information than a nurse or midwife with a fetoscope listening through contractions, and have not been demonstrated to improve birth outcomes. They *are* however, associated with higher cesarean rates.[16] The National Centre for Health Services Research (U.S.) announced in 1978 that "electronic fetal monitoring may do more harm than good."[17] Why then have they been moved from the high risk population they were designed for into the normal labour room?

The list goes on. It is the unfortunate consequence of routine medical intervention that one action leads to the next, in a domino effect. The woman who gets a relatively innocuous intravenous drip "just-in-case" when she arrives in hospital will probably be immobilized flat on her back, thus prolonging her labour. So she is also likely to get an oxytocin hormone drug in her I.V. to speed up the labour. Then an epidural for the unmanageable pain of hormone-stimulated contractions. Next a forceps delivery because the epidural dulls her urge to push. And of course a large episiotomy to make way for the forceps. Her baby may be depressed from the drugs, so it will be taken away to neonatal intensive care for observation. Bonding and breastfeeding are interrupted. The "just-in-case" obstetrical imperative has exposed mother and child to a chain reaction of probably unnecessary risks and traumas. The mother is then congratulated on her "natural birth."

The chain of interventions that distort normal childbirth has many links, and even the medical literature often admits that most of them are weak ones. The following chart describes one of the most common series of events, and the multiplying consequences of the interventions.

It must be emphasized that each intervention has its place, but that is usually in high risk obstetrics, and *only* after its benefits have been scientifically demonstrated. A British study over a decade ago warned that the vast majority of medical interventions are not evaluated by randomized controlled trials.[19] This criticism has not yet been adequately addressed.

Midwives do advocate the use of interventions. They transfer about ten percent of home birth clients to hospital in order to take advantage of obstetrical expertise and tools. But more often, of late, their role is to protect hospital birthing clients from the routine applications of inappropriate intervention. Therein lies the improved safety margin of a hospital birth when a midwife stands by the parents' side.

CHAIN OF EVENTS DISTORTING CHILDBIRTH

Intervention	Routine administration of intravenous fluids.	Confinement to bed.	Stimulation with oxytocin or amniotomy.	Use of analgesics anesthesia.	Use of forceps.	Supine-Lithotomy position.	Episiotomy.
Why?	Because of use of general anesthesia in delivery.	For women with cardiac and respiratory problems only.	Only when medically indicated (e.g. atonic uterus).	Substituted for emotional support from family. Used when medically indicated (e.g. prolonged labor).	For complicated or active management of birth by obstetrician.	Result of developing a table with stirrups and using forceps for delivery. Lack of patience in waiting out the course of labor and of training in basic comfort measures to comfort women and facilitate second stage of labor.	
Consequences	Adds to pathologic environment. Eliminates need for liquid food by mouth. Precipitates metabolic acidosis.	Slows down engagement of fetal presenting part. Decreases maternal circulation. Leads to postural hypotension. Promotes mother waiting for each contraction (no distractions). Reduces effectiveness of contractions.	Elicits stronger, longer contractions with shorter relaxation periods between, making labor process difficult for mother to cope. Presents risk of possible cerebral ischemia and birth trauma for fetus.	Produces lethargic mother who is unable to respond actively to the labor process and narcotized infant with possible respiratory and neurological complications.	Necessitates lithotomy position and episiotomy. May lead to possible damage of infant's facial nerve or brachial plexus or involuntary efforts to expel infant. Increases tension of perinatal tissues. May lead to supine hypotension with resulting decrease of oxygen to fetus.	Requires mother to move at difficult time from labor room to delivery room to maintain sterile field. Necessitates at least local anesthesia. Initiates painful postpartum recuperation, thus leading to more pain medication.	Requires strapping mother to table and shaving perineum to maintain sterile field.

The Stance of the Medical Establishment

Provincial regulatory bodies for physicians, and the various medical associations, appear to be generally opposed to the development of midwifery in Canada. But their opposition is not usually voiced on the basis of safety. Critics of these powerful medical bodies suggest that economic territorialism is the main motivation for keeping midwives out of the system. Kinder observers reflect that the Canadian medical profession is still largely ignorant of the functions and advantages of midwifery. "The doctors are quite sincere," offers a foreign-trained midwife who heads a B.C. obstetrical nursing team, "but they are also sincerely wrong."

This naivete about what midwifery offers is reflected by the commonly used argument that we don't need midwives because we are lucky enough to have lots of doctors. Correspondence from the Quebec Physicians Corporation reflects this presumption: "There is sufficient manpower in the medical profession in Quebec. . .sufficiently well distributed, to handle the delivery of babies."[20] What about woman power?

When the British Columbia Medical Association ruled in 1980 that creating a new profession of nurse-midwives would be "a regressive measure," BCMA President Mel Petreman made this revealing statement: "[Midwifery] is only one tentacle of a thrust in the direction to take over general practice." His colleagues also expressed concern about "two competing services."[21] Clearly it is the role of these bodies to protect the interests of the medical profession first and then to serve public interest.

The Deputy Registrar of the B.C. College of Physicians and Surgeons, C.R. Arnold, writes that practising lay midwives are contravening the Medical Practitioners Act and are therefore liable to prosecution for practising medicine without a license. While other medical bodies hold similar views, no such charges have held against lay midwives. Even when a mortality provides an opening for criminal prosecution, medical experts have failed to convince judges, coroners or juries that the midwives' practices were unsafe or negligent. The recent charges and inquests against midwives have all been initiated by medical personnel, not parents. The medical bodies are clearly unhappy about the emergence of a new class of lay health caregivers who operate outside the reach of medical jurisdiction.

Current medical response to midwifery is intertwined with the home birth safety controversy. In several provinces doctors are effectively prohibited by their colleges from attending home births. Thus the midwives are deprived of on-the-spot medical back-up. This policy is clearly couched in rhetoric about safety, but the "evidence" the colleges put forth falls far short of proof that hospital is safer than home.

The College of Physicians and Surgeons of Ontario, in its position paper *Out of Hospital Births*, quotes out-of-context British statistics: "The perinatal mortality rate for home deliveries in Great Britain is more than 60% higher than the overall rate." Were this in fact the case, one would support inflammatory judgements such as this one from the American College of Obstetrics & Gynaecology: "Home birth is an anti-intellectual, anti-science revolt. . .by the nihilists who want no prenatal care. Home delivery is maternal trauma and child abuse."[22]

When a former British midwife wrote to the Royal College of Obstetrics and Gynaecology in London, querying the damning home birth statistic quoted by the Ontario College, she received this reply:

> Amongst the numbers for statistical purposes are included all cases booked for hospital but who have a precipitate labour and the baby is born at home. Also included are all concealed pregnancies which do constitute a high risk group, and a small proportion of what could be referred to as the "lunatic fringe," mothers who despite having high risk pregnancies still insist in having their babies at home. The overall home delivery figures are therefore inflated by these unusual sub-groups. If one looks at the statistics for patients who are booked for home and deliver at home, this being a low risk group, then the perinatal mortality rate is something around 2 per 1000.[23]

Planned, risk-screened home births with experienced midwives consistently produce such impressive outcomes. And these are the only home births that educated parents and midwives in Canada are advocating. Those investigating the safety of home birth should be wary of raw statistics put forth by medical opponents, and incomplete surveys of the home birth literature. Dr. Lewis Mehl's favourable study is the most significant recent scientific contribution. Yet the committee of the Ontario College who developed the position statement *Out of Hospital Births*, somehow neglected to mention the Mehl study.

Scientifically speaking, the home birth safety debate is still open. Dr. Murray Enkin sums up the current balance:

> Some babies will be lost at home that would not be lost in hospital. And vice versa. Tragedies are inevitable sometimes. . . .The overriding factor in favour of hospital is that the risks of hospital birth are socially acceptable, and the risks at home are not. Everyone must make their own value judgement.

Those parents anxious to make informed value judgements might balance the opinions of the medical establishment against some of the evidence to be found in *The Five Standards of Safe Childbearing* and *The Place of Birth*. They might then echo the startled observation of one academic looking into midwifery: The 'scientist' doctors are operating on the basis of ideology, while, ironically, it is people like The Farm midwives who are collecting statistics.

Doctors in Defense of Midwifery

While the governing medical powers may oppose midwifery, a substantial number of individual physicians are enthusiastic about the prospect. They consider midwifery safe, and recognize that it meets public needs that they simply cannot.

A few dozen Canadian doctors have had ample opportunity to assess the value of midwifery care. These physicians, mostly old fashioned family doctors or open-minded young medics, have developed ongoing professional relationships with practising midwives. Some solicited midwives to help them in their home birth practices. Some had midwives thrust upon them by determined patients, and others agreed (sometimes reluctantly) to provide prenatal care and emergency hospital back-up for local midwives doing home births.

Toronto obstetrician Dr. Ray Osborne was on call to several midwives for three years. As the specialist who received their emergency transfers and answered their queries about complications, Dr. Osborne is in a position to make informed critical evaluations of their work. He admits that in spite of their lack of formal training, ''Most of the decisions the midwives have made have been good. I've been surprised. The level of judgement is high.'' Osborne's role as back-up and consultant to the midwives was a difficult one. He had to be responsive to the most informed and demanding birthing parents, under the disapproving gaze of his obstetrical colleagues. But he recognized that his back-up services created a safer birthing option and one that parents had a right to demand.

Dr. Murry Enkin of McMaster Univeristy Medical Centre also has a mutually respectful relationship with the midwifery community. He reflects that there have been instances when he has not felt confident in the competence of individual midwives, but that he has never encountered one who was not genuinely caring. The professionalization of midwifery he envisages will ensure a basic level of skills and competence. The challenge, he points out, is not to lose that vital element of compassion.

Enkin is quick to mention that there are other priorities in birth besides short-term safety, priorities that midwifery can address:

> It is possible to overstress physical safety. It belongs in the context of the whole picture. The value systems of the woman, her own feel-

ings about what is important. The social dimensions of health, the woman's relationship to significant others like her mate and her own mother.

These factors may indirectly affect safety, but they are also of intrinsic significance. Doctors like Enkin believe that the woman, and the family, have a right to their preferred experience, so long as it is not at odds with the child's best interests. Hospital regulations rarely allow for meeting a woman's individual needs. At this level, he sees "so many holes in the system that you don't know which ones need filling first."

Obstetrician Bernd Wittmann of Vancouver also gives weight to parental satisfaction in his assessment of the efficacy of the pilot midwifery project at the Grace Hospital. While pleased with their safety record, he is most interested to note that:

> the assertive consumers who knew what they wanted. . .emphasized that the most important benefits. . .included the enthusiasm and knowledge of the midwives, the individualized approach to care, the extensive teaching which was part of clinic visits, and the continuous availability of the midwives.[24]

Wittmann sees a clear role for midwives in Canada, because "the average family physician does not have the time to give to the average pregnant family." Also because, in his view, "the situation of obstetrical training for general practitioners in Canada is desperate." After internship some doctors have *seen* as few as 40 births, and the numbers are decreasing in the last few years. Experienced midwives would make more competent experts for normal births.

A further reason for having midwives, former home birth doctor Ben Toane points out, is that they provide home birth care when doctors are not allowed to. "The college has created a demand for midwives," he comments ironically. The Alberta College of Physicians and Surgeons ruled in March 1981 that doctors could not attend home births. Toane was the only physician regularly doing home births in the province at the time. After the ruling the two midwives who worked with him handled deliveries independently. (See Edmonton statistics earlier in this chapter.) As he has done since 1978, Toane continues to provide prenatal and postpartum medical care, and consult with the midwives.

Dr. Toane and Ottawa family physician Gerd Schneider both found midwives indispensable to their home birth practices. Toane admits, "I don't have the patience of a midwife, to sit through entire labours, except for my wife."

"If I were doing it all myself it would be too much," agrees Dr. Schneider. "So the midwife provides good intrapartum care, and calls me when things are imminent. She and the mother handle the delivery. I come just to be there in case they need me."

With a midwife working alongside him, Dr. Schneider feels comfortable taking on two or four home births a month, with a larger hospital clientele. He feels the home birth experience with the midwives benefits his hospital maternity clients. "It is very important for physicians to attend normal, natural births. When they only see complications, they become fearful, which influences a negative attitude toward birth."

He recommends that his hospital clients also work with midwives. "Women with little experience left in a strange environment with their green husbands develop complications. . . .Women with some kind of midwife or coach do better."

"Birth is an experience with the importance of marriage or death," reflects Dr. Schneider. So why should people go through it with so little emotional support? "The midwife's most important function is being with that couple, and that couple *only*."

"Her most important contribution is empathy," echoes Dr. Osborne. Dr. Carmen Price, a general practitioner in Toronto who was called off the home birth front by the College ruling in 1983, describes the midwife's unique contribution as "compassion, something that comes through experience, not through knowledge."

Dr. Price compliments the lay midwives he has worked with for several years on their rare combination of technical skills and caring:

> They have braved all kinds of criticism and legalities to follow a real calling to midwifery. . . .I know what they have done and what they have learned. If I were going to have a baby, I'd have no problem with them, technically, or in any other way. . . .The midwife is vital.

Notes

1.   Doris Haire, "The Cultural Unwarping of Childbirth," in *21st Century Obstetrics Now!* eds. Stewart and Stewart, Mo. 1977, p. 577.
2.   S. Tolagsen, Reporting in *Genesis*, Vancouver, May 1980.
3.   T. Chard and M. Richards eds. *The Benefits and Hazards of the New Obstetrics*, p. 147.
4.   *World Health Statistics,* 1981-81.
     United Nations Demographic Yearbook, 1981.
     United Nations Health Statistics, 1981-82.
     Great Britain Mortality Statistics, 1981.
5.   David Stewart, *The Five Standards for Safe Childbearing*, Mo. 1981, p. 117-118.
6.   Ina May Gaskin, *The Practising Midwife,* Fall 1980, No. 11, pp. 10-11.
7.   L.E. Mehl et al, "Evaluation of Outcomes of Non-Nurse Midwives," *Women and Health,* Summer 1980, pp. 17-23.
8.   L.E. Mehl et al, "Outcomes of Elective Home Births," *Journal of Reproductive Medicine,* November 1977, pp. 281-90.
9.   S. Pullen, Compiled Statistics Dec. 1980 - Dec. 1983, Personal Correspondence, June 7, 1984.

10. Lesley Weatherston et al, "Statistics for the Low Risk Clinic, Grace Hospital," April 1984.
11. David Stewart, "Good Nutrition: The First and Fundamental Standard," in *The Five Standards for Safe Childbearing,* pp. 101-110.
12. Roberto Sosa et al, "The Effect of a Supportive Companion on Perinatal Problems, Length of Labour and Mother-Infant Interaction," *The New England Journal of Medicine.* September 11, 1980.
13. Doris Haire, "The Cultural Unwarping of Childbirth," p. 570.
14. M.E. Stratmeyer, "Research in Ultrasound Bioeffects," *Birth and the Family Journal,* Vol. 7:2, pp. 92-100.
15. R. Caldero-Barcia, "Some Consequences of Obstetrical Interference," *Birth and the Family Journal,* Vol. 2:2 (Reprint).
16. A. Havercamp et al, "The Evaluation of Continuous Fetal Heart Rate Monitoring in High-Risk Pregnancy," *American Journal of Obstetrics and Gynaecology,* Vol. 125, 1976, pp. 310.
17. B.K. Rothman, *In Labor: Women and Power in the Birthplace,* p. 45.
18. S.F. Anderson, "Childbirth as a Pathological Process: An American Perspective," *American Journal of Maternal and Child Health,* Vol. 2, 1977, p. 240.
19. Iain Chalmers, "Implications of the Current Debate on Obstetric Practice," *The Place of Birth,* eds. S. Kitzinger, and J.A. Davis, p. 50.
20. Jacques Briere, Asst. Secretary General, Corporation Professionelle des Medicins du Quebec, Personal Correspondence, February 3, 1984.
21. *Midwifery is a Labour of Love,* Maternal Health Society, p. 94.
22. W.H. Pearse, Editorial, *ACOG Newsletter,* July 1977, p. 3.
23. R.D. Atlay, Honorary Secretary, Royal College of Obstetricians and Gynaecologists, Correspondence with R. Porteous, June 15, 1983.
24. B.K. Wittmann et al, "Hospital-Based Midwifery Care Preliminary Results," Presented at Annual Meeting of Society of Obstetrics and Gynaecology, Vancouver, June 1983.

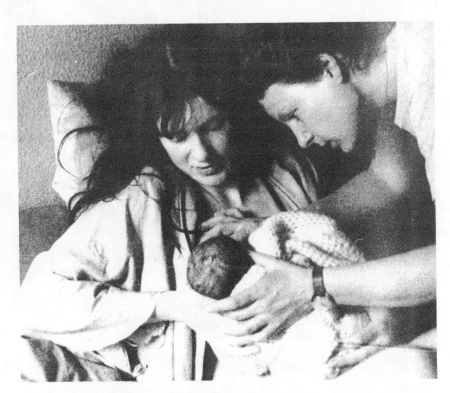

Midwife Sue Rose helps mother and baby establish breastfeeding.

E. Barrington

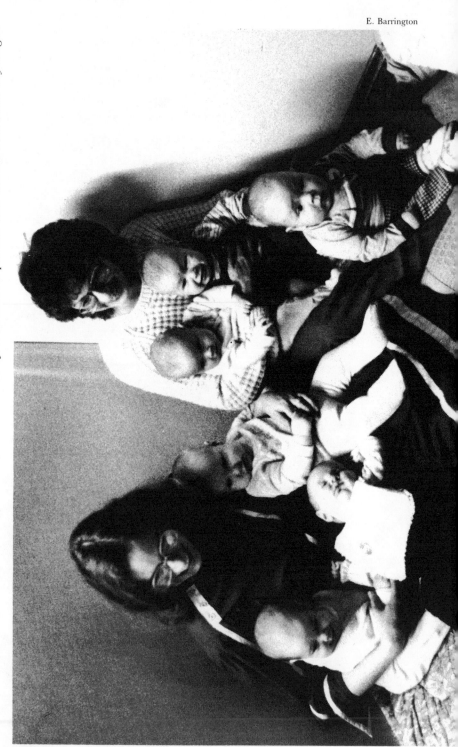

Edmonton midwives Sandy and Noreen at prenatal class reunion with babies they caught.

Chapter Nine

The Law, The Midwifery Movement and The Feminist Alliance

About two years ago, one of our midwives was on her way to a prenatal class on one of the small islands, when the ferry captain came over and said, ''I thought I should warn you that there is somebody on the ferry who told me that he is a detective doing surveillance on you.''

For the next six months, we were operating on paranoia 99% of the time. It became very difficult for our mothers to call us up and say, ''I'm in labour, come to my house,'' because we assumed our phones were being tapped. We devised an intricate system to communicate. There were dogs whelping for six months in Victoria. At three o'clock in the morning.

Then we found out that the detective was investigating a whiplash claim for the Insurance Corporation of British Columbia.[1]

Luba Lyons, Victoria

Is Midwifery Legal?

Canadian midwives practice in an insecure legal limbo. The possibility of prosecution is a nagging threat to all who offer birthing services without benefit of official status. Such paranoia as Lyons described among British Columbia midwives is not entirely un-called for. The persecution of many American midwives who were charged, fined, even imprisoned, for their work[2] reminds their Canadian sisters not to be naive about the legal-political climate in which they operate.

Parents, as well as midwives, are understandably concerned about potential legal liabilities involved in the midwifery care option. ''Is midwifery legal in Canada?'' is the constant question.

The question is not easily answered, because the legal parameters of midwifery practice differ from province to province. As Monique Begin, then Minister of National Health-Welfare, took pains to point out when the issue arose in Parliament in 1984: ''The recognition of midwifery is totally a provincial matter — totally.'' So is the prosecution of midwifery.

There are two charges that midwives fear: one is negligence causing harm or death; the other, practising medicine without a license.

Lawyers, midwives and medical authorities debate about which charge might actually stick — and in which province. Thus far, no practising midwife has been successfully prosecuted on either charge in Canada. (Margaret Marsh, the B.C. woman convicted of practising midwifery in 1980 and fined a token ten dollars, was a former physician and self-described healer, not recognized as a midwife.)[3]

The charge of "practising medicine" is interpreted from those pieces of provincial legislation that give physicians the exclusive right to practise. The viability of a charge depends on the wording of that act. Does it specifically mention "obstetrics" — or even "midwifery" in the definition of practising medicine? Is "midwifery" part of the common law definition of "obstetrics"?

The adjacent chart, summarized from "Midwifery Law: Childbearing Families and the Law Series,"[4] details the relevant Act in every province. It also indicates where provincial licensing bodies for physicians are empowered to license midwives. (Although these powers remain uniformly unexercised.) Almost all provinces do have some provision allowing non-physicians to practise medicine in emergency circumstances, without charge. This provides some legal cover for unpaid midwives.

The charge of criminal negligence can be brought against any individual, but midwives chance it in the everyday course of their work. Conscious that the odds of an unavoidable fatality increase with the number of births they attend, they also recognize that any death in a home birth context is likely to result in legal investigation. Whereas it took 29 suspicious infant deaths at Toronto's Hospital for Sick Children to provoke the Grange Commission, a single death subsequent to a home birth in Halifax in 1983 was cause to charge three midwives with criminal negligence causing death.[5] Although the charges were dropped after a preliminary hearing for lack of evidence of negligence, the three practising midwives in that province were all subjected to ten months of burning at the public stake, between the charge and the dismissal.

In Ontario, the first-ever inquest into a still-birth in hospital was conducted in 1982,[6] because it began as a planned home birth attended by midwives. Although the Ritz baby's death occurred long after arrival at a Kitchener hospital, where there was no qualified doctor present to manage the birth, the midwives suffered the brunt of public scrutiny.

It is important to note that charges against midwives, and the investigations that lead to inquests, have been instigated by reports from medical professionals, not the parents. (Civil medical malpractice suits, on the other hand, only occur when the patient feels wronged.) Usually parents and midwives have presented a unified front in the courts, often sharing the same lawyers. No parent has denounced or regretted their choice of midwifery care when questioned by the courts. Even in the Halifax case, a cause of some concern because the parents' lawyer would not permit them to communicate with the midwives during the course of the action, private testimony from the mother set midwife Donna Marie Carpenter aglow with pride.

The likeliness of a charge against parents subsequent to a midwifery-related tragedy seems remote in Canada at this time. Public reaction to charges against bereaved parents would surely be strong, and likely backfire on the intentions of medical authorities. The available targets for current persecution are those doctors who refuse to conform to medical customs (by backing midwives and attending home births), and the midwives themselves, who dare to operate outside of the medical system.

Parents may ultimately be liable to criminal charges, in the opinion of lawyer Michael Code, who represented David and Andrea Steell at a Toronto inquest into their still-birth at home in 1982.[7] (Both a midwife and a doctor were present at the birth.) Current legal debate about the rights of mothers versus their unborn children is cause for concern. Could a mother be charged for her choice of childbirth attendant on grounds that it contravened the fetus' rights?[8] So is the recent practice in Great Britain of charging fathers and fining them fifty pounds for attending their own children's births, without medical assistance.[9] (Home birth midwifery services are now impossible to find in many parts of Britain.) These fines have been levied in several instances where the birth outcomes at home were excellent.

Although no midwife and no parent in Canada has yet been fined, found guilty or imprisoned in connection with the choice of a birth alternative, several families and midwives have endured the expense and emotional stress of legal proceedings. They all echo that a charge or inquest can be as devastating as a conviction. The scrutiny of press and public and the political machinations drastically alter their lives.

But the gray cloud of the law threatening the midwifery movement has its silver lining. Each ruling that would curtail the practise of midwifery, each charge or inquest, has inadvertently heightened the profile and public support of the midwifery cause. The immediate threat always provokes midwives and parents into more sophisticated political action, and legal proceedings have in fact served to fuel the movement.

LEGAL STATUS OF (NON-PHYSICIAN) MIDWIVES IN CANADA

Province or Territory	Relevant Legislation	Definition of Practising Medicine	Delegated Powers Re: Midwives	Licensing, Legal Status of Practising Midwives
Newfoundland (& Labrador)	*Midwifery Act* c.235, s.3, s.5(1), s.10			Midwives licensed by Newfoundland Midwifery Board. Legal. Few midwives currently licensed.
Nova Scotia	*Medical Act* s.1(d)(c), s.13, s.37(i), s.40(1)(a)(b), s.40(2).	Includes obstetrics but no mention of midwifery.	College of Physicians not authorized to issue any special licenses to midwives.	No mechanism for licensing. Legal/illegal status debatable.
New Brunswick	*Medical Act* 1958. c.74, s.2(1)(c)(d)(e), s.24(1)(a)(b), s.26(k).	A provision states that restrictions on practising medicine do not apply to midwives attending confinements.		No regulation or licensing requirements. No restrictions on midwifery practice. Not illegal.
Prince Edward Island	*Medical Act* M-8, S.27, S.29 (2), S.43.	Undefined. Interpreted therefore as common law definition, likely to include obstetrics.	College not authorized to issue special licenses.	No mechanism for licensing. Legal/illegal status debatable.
Quebec	*Medical Act* c.46, s.1(c)(d), s.29, s.19(a), s.41(c).	Includes attendance at confinements.	Bureau of Physicians may regulate study & practice of obstetrics by midwives. Has never drafted such regulations.	Likely illegal.
Ontario	*Health Disciplines Act* 1974. c.47, s.1.(e), s.45(1) (b), s.50, s.52(1) (a).	Includes obstetrics but the word midwifery removed at last revision.	Council of the College of Physicians can regulate and license midwives. Has not done so.	Legal/illegal status debatable.

	Statute	Definition	Registration	Legal Status
Manitoba	*Medical Act* S.M. 1964. c.29.s.1, s.2(2), s.3, s.14(2), s.32, s.46	Includes the word midwifery.		No provision for licensing or elective practice of midwifery. Probably illegal.
Saskatchewan	*Medical Professions' Act* M-10,s.2, s.28(1), s.29, s.59, s.70(a)(i), s.75.	Defined by statute to include midwifery.		Likely illegal.
Alberta	*Medical Professions' Act* 1975 c.26. s.1(a)(d)(e), s.18(2), s.23(1) (2)(3), s.26(1), s.64(1)(a), (4), s.66(1).	Includes practise of obstetrics.	Council of the College of Physicians may keep special register for midwives. No midwives are on the Special Register.	Unlicensed midwife may practise where there is no registered practitioner. Otherwise legal/illegal status debatable.
British Columbia	*Medical Practitioners' Act.* c.254,s.71, s.72, s.74, s.84.	Includes midwifery.	Council of the College of Physicians determines qualifications for registration. Has not registered any midwives.	Likely illegal.
North West Territories	*Medical Profession Ordinance* M-10, s.2(b), s.3, s.12, s.13, s.33(1)(b)(i).	Includes obstetrics.	To register a practitioner must qualify for registration in a province. No midwives so registered.	Legal/illegal status debatable.
Yukon Territory	*Medical Profession Ordinance* R.O.A58. c.73, s.2(1), 2.8, s.9(1), s.12(1), s.20(1)(b)(j).		To register, a practitioner requires degree from approved medical school.	Legal/illegal status debatable.

The Canadian Midwifery Movement

The political activities of the midwifery community (which includes doctors, prenatal educators, feminists, health professionals and parents), are a direct response to the legal non-status of midwifery in Canada. Midwifery is a political issue and a movement as well as a practice, because it is a freedom curtailed by the legally held monopoly of our medical institutions.

The organized midwifery movement, like the practice of midwifery, developed first in British Columbia. In 1976, a subcommittee of the Maternal Health Society initiated the Campaign Association for the Legalization of Midwifery (CALM). This organization operated quietly for several years, until it sponsored a conference in Vancouver called "Midwifery is a Labour Of Love" in 1981. The conference brought together for the first time practising midwives, and qualified nurse and certified midwives living in British Columbia. The resulting dialogue gave strength and purpose to both groups. This was the intention of CALM conference organizer Karen May, a British Certified Canadian midwife. May is the persistent engineer of unity among B.C. midwives. Midwife Patty Mayr, who had attended about three hundred births in British Columbia at the time of the conference recalls its effect:

> The impetus for political change came from midwives who had been practising in other countries, who were used to being respected . . .and paid. They couldn't handle operating illegally.
>
> At the conference we (practising midwives) suddenly felt more self-respect, and more respect for the profession. Lay midwives who had previously been apologizing for their experience realized that they had attended as many births as some of the doctors. "Hey, wait," we said. "We don't have to beg for respect. We deserve more than this."

Until that point, many of the new midwives had been content to quietly do their work, and to avoid legal controversy as best they could. But due to legal, financial and emotional pressure, the midwife burn-out rate was too high. The most experienced midwives kept retiring.

The Labour Of Love conference, attended by three hundred people, culminated in a mandate to form the Interdisciplinary Midwifery Task Force (MTF) of British Columbia and the Midwives Association of B.C. It sent emissaries out into the international midwifery community, and spread ripples of political awareness to midwifery groups across Canada. The MTF set the agenda for the 1980s — the legalization of a unified midwifery profession, province by province.

The presence of a handful of doctors at subsequent MTF meetings reinforced the self image of the practising midwives. "The doctors wanted to be in on it," Patty Mayr realized. "They must think that something is really happening. . .that this isn't just a ladies' tea party."

The MTF made midwifery legislation for the province its primary goal. Three Victoria midwives proceeded to draft a bill that lawyers pronounced one of the most sophisticated legal documents written by lay people.

Three-time midwife's client and home birth parent Louise Mangan stepped up to be provincial organizer for the MTF. She and other committed consumers and professionals initiated dialogue with government officials and medical bodies and provided a media voice for the midwives. (At the time most practising midwives were still reluctant to come out of the closet for fear of prosecution.)

The midwives formed the Midwives' Association of British Columbia as a professional forum. "Ma B.C." members set to work defining what midwifery meant to them, and discussing how standards of practice might be set. Midwives around the province began to communicate more regularly. Their sisterhood gained strength, although solidarity could not always be maintained among midwives whose practices differed so widely.

Meanwhile Ontario midwife Ava Vosu had been travelling and studying midwifery in the United States. Her political awareness heightened by what she saw there, Ava returned to encourage her Ontario colleagues to create an organization. In spring of 1981, they formed the Ontario Association of Midwives (OAM). This alliance of midwives and public supporters was reinforced by a newsletter *Issue*, that communicated midwifery news across the province.

Following the B.C. example, the OAM mounted a conference in August 1981. Word about this "Loving Hands" conference, to be held in a park near Guelph, went out through developing networks. Speakers from across Canada and the U.S. were invited. In spite of the inevitable Canadian mail strike, close to 75 participants arrived for a five-day midwifery camp. Midwives and parents with infants in arms shared birth stories and sang together under the stars. They attended midwifery skills workshops and discussed political strategy. Ontario midwives were strengthened by contact with politically experienced colleagues from the United States. The conference energized them to face adversity to come.

Subsequent conferences were held in British Columbia, Ontario, and other provinces, importing internationally respected professionals to lend credence to the local midwifery cause. At various times Sheila Kitzinger of Britain's National Childbirth Trust, Holland's Professor G.J. Kloosterman, the former head of the International Federation of Gynaecology & Obstetrics, Dorothea Lang of the International Childbirth Education Association, and David Stewart, of NAPSAC International, all came to Canadian conferences. Their credentials, statistics and experience contributed to the case for legalizing midwifery in Canada.

Conferences, along with the various midwives' and consumer organizations with their newsletters, became the primary vehicles of the midwifery movement. Whenever legal or political events posed a threat to midwifery practice, these organizational machines informed the public, alerted the media, and rallied supporters into action.

Courts and College Rulings as Catalysts

Legal proceedings, and the rulings of medical authorities intended to curtail midwifery practice, have provoked increasingly sophisticated organization in the midwifery movement.

The medical bodies that most often threaten midwifery are the provincial Colleges of Physicians & Surgeons. They are empowered to govern and license doctors, and have no overt interest in midwifery, except where it is perceived as encroaching on the practice of medicine. They do, however, have jurisdiction over the doctors who cooperate with midwives, and those who attend home births.

Midwives need good professional relationships with doctors to practise optimally. They require medical consultation in emergencies, second opinions in the course of prenatal care, and because midwives have no status in hospital, they must arrange doctor back-up for hospital transfers. Where midwives are forced to practise without good doctor and hospital relations, attendance at home births involves higher risks, and attendance at hospital births can become a political battle.

Politicization of the B.C. midwives began back in 1976, when the two doctors who were regularly attending home births both lost their privileges at St. Paul's Hospital, the preferred maternity venue. The charges against them were unrelated to home birth attendance, which was medically acceptable practice. But the timing and coincidence could not be ignored. Nor could subsequent pressure on other doctors in the province to stop providing prenatal care or back-up to mothers planning home births with midwives. Practising midwives began to slowly acknowledge the power plays they were caught up in. Parents got angry about being denied medical care.

The Alberta College of Physicians and Surgeons challenged the midwifery and home birth movement in that province onto its feet in March of 1981. It banned doctor attendance at home births,[10] a unique move in Canada. Displaying the depth of his concern for the public, College

Registrar Dr. Roy Le Riche was quoted in *Calgary Magazine*, January 1982 as saying, "We don't care if mothers have their babies in manure piles at home, as long as they don't involve the medical profession."

The Calgary Association of Parents and Professionals for Safe Alternatives in Childbirth (CAPSAC), existing in various forms since 1975, incorporated legally as an affiliate of the powerful U.S.-based lobby organization NAPSAC. The Edmonton Association for Safe Alternatives in Childbirth (ASAC), formed in 1979, responded by stepping up political activity. Edmonton was most affected by the College ruling because the two midwives practising there had been attending all births with Dr. Benjamin Toane. (The ruling was aimed directly at Dr. Toane as the only Alberta physician regularly doing home births at the time.) Ironically, the Edmonton midwives became independent birth attendants as a result of that College ruling.

The Alberta College ruling made the national press, and provoked editorials and letters-to-the-editor in Alberta papers. The Alberta birth alternatives groups gained membership. The midwives of the province got together to form the Alberta College and Register of Domicilliary Midwives Association (ACRDMA), and pursued legalization of their profession. With no doctors doing home births, demand for midwifery services increased.

When the Alberta Health Occupations Board (HOB) commenced hearings in 1983, ACRDMA was ready to present a strong case for a midwifery profession. Dr. Le Riche of the College sent notice to the Board that legalizing midwifery "would be going back to the dark ages. . .a retrograde step."[11] But CAPSAC and ASAC researched and presented a well-documented brief, reinforced by articulate parent interviews. The Board responded quite favourably, as midwife-presenter Sandra Botting relates: "A member of the Board in a wheelchair came up to me afterward and told me that if *he* were having a baby, he'd have it at home with me attending. I had to tell him that he'd be too high risk!"

The HOB exercise was not expected to win immediate results, and in fact the midwifery proposal was turned down. However, the HOB encouraged ACRDMA to seek an alliance with nurse-midwives and then return with a proposal for a unified midwifery rather than domicilliary midwifery profession.[12]

As a public relations strategy, the HOB application served the Alberta midwifery movement well. Reactionary statements from the College of Physicians and Surgeons fanned the fervour of both parents and public.

In Ontario, the first formal challenge to the nascent Ontario Association of Midwives was the Ritz baby inquest in Kitchener in May-June 1982. The summer 1982 *Issue* reports that:

> The inquest has played a key role in bringing together the midwives of Southern Ontario. Many of us have finally begun to meet en masse with the doctors who support home birth. . . .In Toronto some of the nurses and midwives have begun to talk about our role as labour coaches (in the hospital). The OAM has now selected officers to carry out the tasks of a very active organization.

The OAM retained prominent lawyer Clayton Ruby for the inquest. Legal costs posed the first hurdle, so a letter to former midwives' clients soliciting $50 donations was mailed out. With no tax deduction to promise, and only a subscription to *Issue* as concrete return, that one letter netted $10 thousand in donations. Along with the money arrived sheaves of personal support letters, to be presented to the C.P.S.O. at a politically opportune moment.

Although press coverage was not always favourable or accurate, and the inquest findings not in keeping with the assessment of expert witnesses like Dr. Murray Enkin, the final message was clear: Coroner Jack Burger recommended licensing and standards for midwives in Ontario. He hoped that communication between doctors, nurses and midwives would be improved, adding regretfully that:

> It's not my experience of the College of Physicians and Surgeons that they take a broadminded view on too many new or controversial matters. After all, the College is pretty rigid — they've preached defensive medicine all down the line.[13]

The machinery of the Ontario midwifery movement was well oiled when a second inquest occurred in Toronto in August of that same summer. Although a home birth doctor, rather than the midwife, would take the weight of responsibility in the Steell baby inquest, the OAM provided support for midwife, doctor and parents. Midwives by then understood that progressive doctors needed political help almost as much as they did.

During the inquest, the courtroom was crammed with mothers, some breastfeeding their babies. Coroner Paul Tepperman remarked on the good behaviour of the babies, appreciating their occasional "editorial comments" — gurgles and squeals.[14] The verdict of the coroner's jury on July 14 recommended standards for home births, and the training and accreditation of birth coaches.

While raising the midwifery issue in the context of the few rare instances of death is always unfortunate, these two inquests did reinforce the midwives' demands for acknowledged status that would allow them formal training. Both inquest rulings directed the health and medical authorities to make a place for midwives. Both inquests contributed the necessary media attention to educate the public about the existence of midwives and the need for them. They also deepened the ties between pro-midwifery organizations across Canada and the U.S. In Fall of 1982, all the international subscribers to *NAPSAC News* received an issue headlined "Midwifery on Trial in Canada." In unity, the midwifery movement found new financial, moral and political strength.

In 1983, the OAM received an indirect challenge from the College of Physicians and Surgeons. A policy statement on "Out of Hospital Births," accompanied by not-so-well veiled threats to individual physicians, effectively reduced the number of physicians attending home births in Toronto from seven to one within six months. Since the Toronto midwives were only attending home births in conjunction with these physicians, the College ruling placed them in a new position of legal vulnerability. Parents who wanted doctors as well as midwives at their home births were outraged. A new consumer organization called Choices in Childbirth mounted a much-publicized week long demonstration in front of the C.P.S.O. building.

Attending births on their own for the first time, the Toronto midwives gained new confidence in their professional abilities. They requested and received more political support from the parents they served. The College ruling was one factor in the formation of the Midwifery Task Force of Ontario in the Fall of 1983. This MTF would take some of the political work off the overburdened midwives' shoulders. They could step back now, to let parents and supporters help organize fund-raising events, letter campaigns, political lobbying, and media liaison.

Another indication of the political maturation of the midwifery movement was the fact that Toronto midwives were already coming forward. They realized that in order to be treated as legitimate professionals, they had to represent themselves openly as such.

> The authorities certainly know who we are. The public needs to know too, so they will recognize and defend us when we need them. . . .A lot of our cover is in being out front, in declaring our occupation as "midwife."
>
> — Jane Cocks

But midwives were only able to "come out" when public support for their cause was strong enough to offset the likeliness of prosecution. A lone midwife without consumer and media support was still a sitting duck across most of the country. Saskatchewan midwives, for instance, did not feel that their "birth base" was large enough to defend them, even in 1984. They remained rumoured first names, to be found via protective networks.

The theory of court case as catalyst to the movement held one more time in Halifax in 1983. In the Atlantic provinces, where midwifery previously had little impact, charges against Halifax midwives provoked new awareness and support. The tiny local birth alternatives group, unable to cope with the financial stress of criminal proceedings, reached out across Canada, and to NAPSAC and the Alternative Birth Crisis Coalition (A.B.C.C.) in the United States. Their case became a national media event, and A.B.C.C. president Marion Thompson (also a founder of the La Leche League) flew to Halifax to face the media with the midwives.

The case culminated in full exoneration of the midwives. It spawned a Nova Scotia NAPSAC chapter, complete with newsletter. The Midwifery Coalition of Nova Scotia, active in three cities, developed next. The newly-activated birthing community made presentations to the Legislative Select Committee on Health, and The National Task Force on The Allocation of Health Care Resources.[15] Following her ten month ordeal with the law, midwife Donna Marie Carpenter emerged with new confidence and political purpose: "I feel totally renewed. We're not going to let it go. We're going to do all the groundwork. I'm going to work on midwifery legislation."

Parents as Activists

Birth has such a powerful personal impact that when authorities impose restrictions on people's birth plans, they are often provoked to political action. Even those who have never previously found cause to question authority will turn militant when they feel their childbirth rights infringed upon.

Parents are shocked and angered when they discover how little power and status they have when confronted by medical institutions and authorities. University professor Allan Cheyne recalls how appalled he was at being excluded from the cesarean birth of his daughter: "They locked me out! It was a violation of my rights — not just as a father, but as a human being." He moved his family across the province to ensure a midwife-attended birth for the next child.

Alberta parents called in the Civil Liberties Association over the ruling that prohibited doctors from attending home births.[16] The Kootenay Parents' group in British Columbia challenged the B.C. College on its policy of withdrawing prenatal care from mothers planning home births. The Deputy Registrar of the College was unapologetic: "An individual or family has no 'right' to the provision of any kind of medical service from a licensed medical doctor, if that doctor is of the opinion that the requested service is not in the best interest of the patient or offspring."[17]

This statement excused publicly paid doctors for denying care to home birth parents, although home birth has never been proven less safe than hospital. However, mothers who posed *proven* safety threats to their unborn — smoking, drinking, taking drugs, or not eating adequately — were never denied medical care.

Denial of parents' rights, as much as loyalty to the midwives, has created the consumer strength of the midwifery movement in the 1980s. Parents swell the demonstrations and fan the flames of media interest. In April 1983 *Toronto Star* journalist Michele Landsberg declared that she could never print the volume of reader response to a column on midwifery. Producers of a TV Ontario phone-in show felt obliged to write to health authorities when a programme on midwifery provoked their highest-ever audience reaction. During the show, 1,700 callers voted nine to one in favour of legalizing midwifery in the province.[18]

When parents began to take a political stand, the movement made a quantum leap, and the midwives breathed deep sighs of relief. It is very difficult to be a good midwife and a good politician at the same time. Consumer activists have lessened the burden of these contradictory imperatives on Canadian midwives.

Political Progress

The midwifery movement has had many setbacks and suffered occasional losses of impetus, but it has nevertheless gained much ground since 1972. The first political step was simply using the word "midwife" in Canada. Then came years of practising openly as a political demonstration. Legal awareness dawned and midwives began signing "Informed Consents" with their clients, delineating responsibilities and clarifying legal risks.

The government of Quebec was the first to show an active interest in institutionalizing midwifery. Officials participated in the 1981 conference *Accoucher ou Se Faire Accoucher* (To Deliver or To Be Delivered). A government report on the potential for midwifery services was subsequently promised. It was to be presented to the Minister of Education and published in 1983. Meanwhile, Naissance-Renaissance (Birth-Rebirth), the organization supporting midwifery founded in 1981, received funding for film projects, staff, and even a slick magazine, *L'Une A L'Autre*.

But the report was never released. Perhaps the medical lobby intervened? Perhaps the government did not perceive sufficient public demand for midwifery?

What the Quebec movement lacks, the midwives speculate, is a corps of committed volunteers like the parent activists who pressure other provincial governments. French Quebec has no tradition of voluntarism, they suggest.

Although demand for their services far exceeds their birthing capacity, this demand has not translated itself into public action. Without organized consumer pressure, the initial enthusiasm of the Quebec government was not sustained. And nothing changed.

In provinces where the client base evolved into an active public following, midwives began to strongly influence public opinion in the 1980s. With solid consumer support, they poised for the leap into political forums. Long-time organizer Karen May looks back on the evolution:

> We've been grinding away at changing public attitudes, rather than getting concrete things done. Now we have internal organization, we're learning lobbying.We're psychically ready to make our move — to walk up the steps of parliament.

Ontario midwives did walk up the steps of their legislature in 1984. The NDP tabled a Private Members Bill proposing an independent midwifery profession, covered by the Ontario Health Insurance Plan.[19] Midwives lobbied MPPs, seeking support for the bill, while parents signed petitions proving the voting power of the midwifery lobby.

By Fall 1984, the Ontario Association of Midwives had grown strong enough to mount several simultaneous political actions. The NDP Private Member's Bill dovetailed with the deliberations of the Health Professions Legislative Review Committee, considering the legalization of the profession. A joint OAM, Ontario Nurse-Midwives Association (ONMA), Midwifery Task Force (MTF) submission to this Committee called for a unified profession with a College of Midwives and midwifery school.[20]

To further multiply the impact of the midwifery issue on public, press, legislators and Health Ministry officials, the MTF hosted the Midwives Alliance of North America (MANA) Conference in Toronto that November. International speakers provided a timely amplification of the views of Ontario midwifery advocates, and the recent accreditation of several Canadian midwifery organizations by the prestigious International Confederation of Midwives further strengthened the legitimacy of the case.

The Conservative government blocked the bill, but by then, doctors, hospitals, health officials and even the CSPO were beginning to consider the inevitability of legalized midwifery in Ontario. The movement turned its attention to questions like: What kind of midwifery? How? and When? But before the battle would be won, one further alliance awaited.

Midwifery and Feminism

Legal threats and restrictive rulings uged the midwifery movement into organized action, but a late-blooming alliance with feminism was to provide an essential political power base. In 1984 the concerned constituency swelled from parents and health professionals into the politicized female population.

Some feminist midwives and feminist mothers had cross-pollinated midwifery and the women's movement from the start, but the groups historically viewed each other with mutual suspicion. No wonder: The feminism of the early 1970s was engaged in freeing women from the shackles of childbirth and mothering. Feminist writers like Shulamith Firestone actually called for technological reproduction. The new midwifery meanwhile celebrated those very biological differences.

Although the women's movement created the confidence that allowed midwifery to flourish, and midwifery was a practical example of a woman-centred system, many feminists were ill-at-ease with counterculture midwives. And midwives couldn't embrace a women's movement that appeared to reject motherhood. Assumptions about the abortion issue created a further wedge between the two movements.

The mutual interests of midwifery and feminism were evident to some women all along. Vicki van Wagner chose midwifery as her profession precisely because it offered her an avenue for feminist action. Some of her colleagues came to midwifery from politically-motivated women's self-health groups. Others became feminists as a result of their experiences as midwives. Clients' stories of oppression at the hands of male medics tended to repeat an unmistakeable political pattern.

The midwives' legal vulnerability to harassment from medical institutions contributed to their feminist eye-opening. By the late 1970s most midwives were seriously questioning the male authorities who challenged the validity of their vocation.

Mothers, too, were developing feminist perspectives through midwifery. Holly Nimmons of the Midwifery Task Force of Ontario describes the feminist awakening she hears told so often:

> It is a powerful experience as a woman to be supported by other women in such a dramatic event as giving birth. It is even more impressive to realize the vast difference in care between a female midwife and a male doctor. Seeing their needs better served, midwives' clients learn to look more to other women for support.

Often a midwife is a middle-class mother's first accessible, acceptable model of that foreign species of woman called "feminists." Meeting fellow clients who share her concerns about securing childbirth choices, the young mother finds herself poised to act on other women's behalf.

The midwifery movement has provided a comfortable forum for many a new feminist's first tentative political steps.

Mothers and midwives together matured politically in response to adversity. As the clientele broadened and ambitions for legalization deepened, the concepts of compromise and alliance increasingly appealed. Certainly a few religious midwives of the anti-abortion stance would never embrace feminism, but by the 1980s, most of the midwifery movement was ready to join forces with a feminism that declared itself "Pro-Choice, Pro-Baby."

The women's movement was also evolving. Feminist sociologist Mary O'Brien recalls a change of heart among her colleagues in the mid-seventies, exemplified by her own eye-opening experience. Along with a group of women activists, she set out into the Toronto suburbs to build support. They were surprised to discover that their condescending attitude toward "housewives" was mirrored back. "Without having children," O'Brien realized, "our claim to represent femininity was spurious."

The feminism of the latter 1970s shifted its focus from "making it in a man's world" to "making a woman's world." Feminists endeavoured to create new structures and support systems to accommodate their particular needs. . .structures like daycare, women's centres and abortion clinics. Motherhood became a chosen option in the emerging woman's world. And midwifery was a new structure to serve feminist mothers.

Suddenly there were many of them. A generation of women activists in their thirties, prompted by the biological alarm clock, chose motherhood, now or never. Instead of a barrier to career advancement, reproduction was now seen as an opportunity to explore the physical and symbolic meaning of being female. Like the midwives, these feminists embraced pregnancy and parenting as women's special strengths.

Among the midwives, feminists found a revival of the lost female birth culture, as well as a truly woman-centred care system. The midwives history, told in books like *Witches, Midwives and Nurses*,[21] was easily recognized as another feminist struggle, and midwifery practice was a symbolic representation of women relying on themselves.

Midwifery could simultaneously validate women's traditional strengths such as nurturing, listening and responding emotionally, while requiring all the powers of the new woman: intellectual decisiveness, independence and ambition. It was women working with and for women, in a specifically female biological and social realm. Caught up in the new 1980s' celebration of motherhood, midwives and feminists finally found each other.

The relationship between the two movements was formalized in 1984, when the National Action Committee on the Status of Women resolved to lobby for legalized midwifery.[22] Gradually, the concept of "choice" was opening up. At first, it had referred to a choice of whether or not to conceive: birth control. Then as a choice of whether or not to carry a pregnancy: abortion. The feminist understanding of the mid-1980s was ready to embrace a concept of choice that included choices in childbirth, particularly midwifery care.

In 1984 the gender lines of the midwifery-versus-medical authority battle were clearly drawn. The Canadian Medical Association reported in 1983 that over 85% of Canadian physicians, and over 90% of obstetricians, were still men. More and more feminists solidified the tardy alliance between midwifery and the women's movement. They recognized, as Mary O'Brien asserts, that, "Midwifery is integral to the women's movement. It is a triumphant affirmation of women's right to choose."

Feminism lent the midwifery movement complex new networks, political savvy, and imposing numerical strength. This alliance catapulted the midwifery issue into mainstream political forums; the public arenas where legalization will eventually be won.

Notes

1. Abridged from *Midwifery Is A Labour Of Love,* Maternal Health Society, p. 30.
2. "Midwifery In Transition," *NAPSAC News,* Vol. 8 No. 2, Summer 1983.
3. R.v. Marsh, Victoria, B.C., 1980. Unreported.
4. "Midwifery Law," *Childbearing Families and the Law Series,* Community Task Force in Maternal and Child Health, Winnipeg, (Health Promotion Directorate. Health and Welfare Canada Project No. 1216-6-132).
5. R.v. Carpenter, MacLellan and Wheelden, Preliminary Hearing, October 25, 26 and November 25, 1983, Halifax, Unreported.
6. Jean Ritz, Inquest, May 20, 21 and June 18, 1982, Kitchener, Ontario, Coroner Jack Burger, Available at Chief Coroner's Office of Ontario.
7. Simon Peter Steell, Inquest, July 12, 13, 14, 1982, Toronto, Coroner P. Tepperman M.D., Available at Chief Coroner's Office of Ontario.
8. Bernstein, Hannah. "Study Urged Into Status of Unborn Child," *Canadian Bar Foundation News,* March 1984, p. 3.
9. "Midwife Father Fined In Scotland," *The Practising Midwife,* Winter 1981.
10. College of Physicians and Surgeons of Alberta, "Resolution Prohibiting Elective Domicilliary Midwifery by a Member" 1981.
11. Mark Tait, "MDs to Battle Bid Allowing Midwives," *Calgary Herald,* Oct. 28, 1982.
12. Sandra Botting, "News Update," *Birth Issues,* Vol. 1, No. 1, Nov., Dec. 1983.
13. Michael Kieran, "Proposal To License Midwives," *The Globe and Mail,* June 25, 1982.
14. Blaise Hopkinson, "Inquest on Baby Death," *Toronto Sun,* July 15, 1982.
15. V. and R. O'Day, *APSAC Nova Scotia Newsletter* #2, February 1984.
16. "The Canadian Charter of Rights and Freedoms Challenge To The College of Physicians and Surgeons," Alberta Civil Liberties Association.

17. C.R. Arnold, corresponding for the British Columbia College of Physicians and Surgeons with M. Jansma, December 14, 1983.
18. M.C. Dufour, T.V. Ontario "Medical Intervention In Childbirth," *Speaking Out*, Produced by Carol Burton-Fripp, First aired Nov. 10, 1983.
19. Bill 48, "An Act to Establish Midwifery as a Self-Governing Profession," Legislature of Ontario, First Reading April 26, 1984.
20. Vicki Van Wagner et al, "Brief on Midwifery Care In Ontario," December 1983.
21. B. Ehrenreich and D. English, *Witches, Midwives and Nurses,* Feminist Press, New York 1983.
22. Resolution 15, "To Support Legalization of Midwifery Services In Canada," National Action Committee on the Status of Women, Passed March 18, 1984, Annual General Meeting, Ottawa.

Mark Laforet

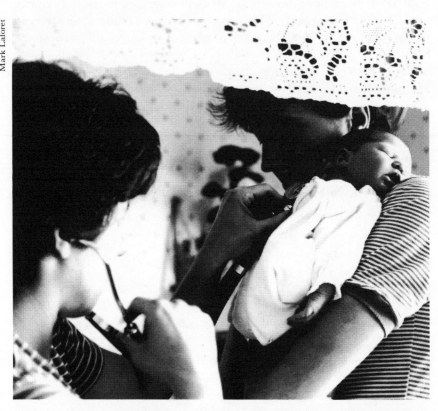

Midwife Gale checks newborn's heartbeat at postpartum visit.

Chapter Ten
Legalization:
Midwifery Meets Medicine

Midwifery is a real need. We are getting into a desperate situation with family doctors opting out of obstetrics. Midwives are the logical and necessary means of filling the gap.

> Dr. Murray Enkin,
> Obstetrician

There's no question. We'll have licensed midwives in the next three to five years.

> Dr. Ray Osborne,
> Obstetrician

Why Legalization is Inevitable

Inside of a decade, the concept of legal midwifery in Canada has transformed from a far-fetched fantasy into an inevitability. Consumer demand and financial strain on the health care system have suggested the need for a midwifery option and, most recently, the exodus of general practitioners from the birthing scene has left a care gap that only midwifes can fill.

Due to time pressure, complex obstetrical procedures, and escalating medical insurance premiums, it is no longer practical or possible for most family doctors to continue attending their patients' births. In response to the growing number and expense of malpractice suits, the Canadian Medical Protective Association has hiked annual insurance rates for GPs attending births from $35 in 1971 to $1,200 in 1984. (General Practitioners not attending births now pay $550.) Few family doctors do enough births in a year to justify this investment, without utterly disrupting their office practices and personal lives. While obstetricians have also experienced an exponential premium increase (from about $35 in 1971 to $1,950 in 1984), their fee base and volume of births still justifies the expense.

Midwifery advocates have sought to broaden, rather than narrow, the carestyle options available to childbirth consumers, so they regret the departure of the GPs from the birthing scene. Many midwives have enjoyed cooperative relationships with family physicians, who understand the midwife's role better than a high risk trained obstetrician. But no one in the midwifery movement doubts that as the GPs opt out of birth, the midwife's political position improves.

Who but midwives will serve all the normal birthing mothers previously attended by their family doctors? Obstetricians? Many wary consumers now know that an obstetrician is not an appropriate caregiver if a natural birth is to follow a normal pregnancy.

> We're not properly trained for normal births. We'd have to learn new skills: how to recognize and support what is normal. But if an obstetrician spends all his time on normal birth, he can't maintain his skills in handling pathology. He's left with the difficult choice of short-changing either the normal or the high risk patient.
>
> — Dr. Murray Enkin

Faced with a growing volume of normal maternity patients with ambitions for natural childbirth, the obstetrician becomes a victim of his very expertise. He is ill-equipped to satisfy his patients, and if he does concede to their demands, he may be subject to the disapproval of his specialist colleagues.

Many obstetricians don't want to do large volumes of normal births. To a highly-trained academic mind, normal is boring, and non-interventive births can be a waste of their education and skills. Nor is there much financial incentive to take over the GP's role. Gynecology is more profitable and less time-consuming than obstetrics. Some specialists basically take on maternity patients as loss leaders, hoping to serve their ongoing gynecological needs.

Since obstetricians are unavailable in parts of the country, ill equipped to handle the demands of the new childbirth consumer, and perhaps unwilling to take over all births, the need for another maternity caregiver becomes plain.

Another catalyst toward legalized midwifery is the current financial crisis of our health care system. Universal tax-supported medicine is threatened, the public purse strings are drawn tight, and yet we continue to support the most expensive style of maternity care, high-tech obstetrics, even where it is neither necessary nor beneficial.

Midwifery is cheaper than obstetrics. Politicians and health bureaucrats can't help but approve it. Two recent studies in the U.S. determined an average savings of $100-800 per birth attended by a midwife rather than an obstetrician.[1] A report to the Registered Nurses Association of British Columbia in 1976 found the cost of management of a pregnancy by an obstetrician to be $630. If a midwife were in charge the figure dropped to $240.[2] A 1972 study by the Canadian Hospital Association, the Canadian Medical Association and the Canadian

Nurses' Association estimated an $8.2 million annual savings at that time, if births were not attended by physicians.[3] These studies do not even begin to tally up the costs of obstetrical technology avoided by midwifery care, nor the savings involved in home, rather than hospital births.

Consumer demand and political pressure are of course the deciding force in favour of midwifery for Canadians. After a decade of public education and media attention on the midwifery cause, it is now understood and advocated by a significant block of parents, feminists and health care professionals. As they translate their opinion into petitions, demonstrations and votes, even the most conservative legislators take note.

In 1984, the care gap left in the wake of opting out GPs, the potential cost savings of a midwifery option, and public pressure all propel us toward legalization of midwifery.

Barriers to Legalization

Research in Canada and the United States has defined several classes of barriers to the institutionalization of midwifery services for Canadians.[4] They are financial, legal, structural and attitudinal.

In spite of the long-term savings to the public purse that midwifery can promise, there are financial barriers such as incorporating payment for midwives' services into provincial health insurance plans. This is essential in order that all classes have fair and equal access to midwives' services. If clients had to pay out-of-pocket as with dentistry services, those most in need would likely go without. The social benefits of midwifery would be minimized.

Clauses 2 and 9 of the amendment to the new Canada Health Act, pushed through by the Canadian Nurses Association in 1984, go a long way to alleviate this obstruction to the institutionalization of universal midwifery care. It requires provincial insurance plans to reimburse not just doctors, but "health care practitioners." Once midwifery becomes a designated health profession in any province, her services will automatically be covered.

Legal barriers to a midwifery system begin with the provincial legislation which currently restricts their practice (see Chapter Nine). All these statutes would have to be rewritten.

Structural barriers include the organization of hospitals and teaching institutions and the current physician supply. How and where would we fit the midwives in? We have no birthing centres, the obvious venue. How fundamentally would hierarchies and systems have to be altered?

Public opinion is another barrier. While an educated vocal minority favours midwifery, the public at large is still in awe of medicine, and not aware of the benefits of midwifery care. Initially, acceptance of a new profession of midwives would have to be enhanced through public education.

But all of these barriers are the kind that governments frequently overcome. Legislators can and do change laws. Health departments mount public education campaigns. Bureaucrats and administrators restructure institutions. It is all possible — with the cooperation of the medical profession.

In fact, the greatest barrier to a midwifery system for Canada has been the powerful medical lobby. Long entrenched in the system, closely allied with governments, well financed for its propaganda war, medicine has ample resources and connections to defend its own professional territory.

Although there are indications of a gradual shift of opinion among the rank and file, the institutions of organized medicine are still solidly opposed to legalizing midwifery. This rejection is couched in considerations of safety and public service, but professional self-interest is readily apparent. At the moment doctors enjoy a monopoly position and unquestioned authority. They have no desire to open the door to a competing philosophy of maternity care. Even as medical authorities begin to concede to the possibility of midwives entering the system, they seek to restrict and define the emerging profession to their own advantage.

Risks of Legalization

One of the greatest religions in the world today is medicine. The same thing could happen to the midwives, if they begin disciplining and defending their own.

— Dr. Carmen Price

Some midwifery advocates do not welcome legalization. Others pursue it with mixed feelings. They foresee the midwife's role co-opted by the system, her philosophy of care corrupted. Pointing to midwifery systems in Europe and the United States that fall far short of current Canadian ideals, they ask if professional midwives will still be able to respond personally to parents' individual needs. Will responsibility to doctors and hospitals who hire them interfere with the primary alliance to clients? Will formal qualifications replace her current striving for up-to-date skills with "qualified" complacency?

They envision midwives working eight-hour shifts in hospital, so that continuity of care is impossible; midwives who take up the profession to make a living rather than follow a calling. Will such women be willing or able to provide the powerful empathy that now distinguishes our midwifery care? And what about midwives tailor-made by the medical system, wooed to embrace high-tech birth? Examining midwifery systems in some European countries, where the profession offers little more than improved safety statistics, all of these qualms become justified concerns.

When legalization has been pursued by the politically naive, the consequences have been appalling and ironic. In California, where the new midwifery first flourished, legal status was achieved at the expense of the very women who re-invented the profession. Nurse-midwifery was instituted and lay-midwifery outlawed. The nurse-midwifery option offered by the system clearly fails to satisfy the public, since lay midwives are still much in demand. But several of those who dare to practise have been fined, charged, and even imprisoned for continuing their work.

It is not inconceivable that compromise legislation in Canadian provinces would commit the same tactical errors. Many of our current lay midwives would remain ''illegals'' if the profession is not so defined as to favour them. If the principles of the new midwifery are not firmly entrenched in the system of regulation we create, we might actually see midwives contributing to the restriction of childbirth options like home birth. There is no reason to believe that midwives are immune to co-optation.

In spite of the potential pitfalls, the midwifery movement is increasingly unanimous in its pursuit of legalization. Most of the reluctant are persuaded by social conscience. How can one conscientiously enjoy the services of a midwife when the majority of the population, including those most in need, are not even aware of her existence? As it is now, only a minority with time, money, and information have access to the few available midwives. The status quo is difficult to justify.

It is also impossible to maintain. Practising midwives are paying a personal price that they cannot sustain for years. No longer can they simply carry on quietly practising, without fear of legal reprisal. Midwifery is out of the closet, and impetus for public acceptance and demand for accessibility is building. Times and circumstances have changed. Opportunities must be seized. Or someone else will seize the opportunity to squash them!

Furthermore, there are weaknesses in the current midwifery practice that only legalization can correct. We have no recognizable standards of practice or means of formal training. Midwives have no status within the hospital, where most women choose to give birth. The lack of medical back-up and cooperation with doctors is a serious safety consideration, particularly in the case of home births.

In other respects, select Canadian families now enjoy a brand of midwifery care that is the envy of the world. The international health community is watching to see if we will manage to preserve the personal, responsive, responsible and exacting midwifery of which we can now boast.

The challenge of legalization is to protect strengths while alleviating weaknesses. The most fearful error is embodied in all the negative connotations of the words "*professional*" and "*institutional*." "Let's continue to strive for organization where uniqueness is encouraged, respected and celebrated," warns midwife-author Elizabeth Davis, "or we will become just another technical profession."[5]

If we fail to protect the true philosophy of the new midwifery, including that individuality, whatever system we create will fail. A new grassroots crop of illegal midwives will emerge in the 1990s, to remind us of the shortcomings of the system. We need more than mere legalization. We need a midwifery service people *like*.

Safeguards for Quality Midwifery

Legalization appears to be an attainable goal in certain provinces. Within a few years Ontario, Alberta or British Columbia will pass the necessary legislation. Presumably, the domino effect will then spread the innovation across the country.

But the kind of midwifery most readily won in the political arena will not necessarily provide the quality of care we now know. Advocates must be careful not to make disastrous compromises in their efforts to hasten legislation. They need to carefully assess various models and options, identifying priorities and safeguards for the kind of midwifery they seek.

Positions and strategies vary from place to place, but certain concepts emerge repeatedly as keys to the preservation of the new midwifery.

The first axiom is that midwives have an independent, self-governing profession. If midwives are subject to professional discipline according to medical standards, rather than midwifery ones, it will be all but impossible for them to provide an alternative — and complement — to medical care. The methods and perspectives of midwifery and medicine are often at odds. The union of these differences serves the consumer, as Dr. Carmen Price illustrates:

> If two doctors, trained the same way, with the same technology and pathology in obstetrics, agree on a cesarean section, then that is better than one doctor.
>
> But when a midwife and I, coming from totally different places, from opposite ends, can agree that a woman needs a section, then you can bet we're dead on. She does.

Placing midwives below doctors on the authority hierarchy would effectively shackle them, but an adversary relationship between the two professions would be equally counterproductive. What the public needs is "Teamwork, . . .the reciprocal appreciation of the skills of others linked together in a unified effort toward a mutual end."[6] This relationship must be nurtured by the governing structures set up in legislation.

Similarly, midwifery cannot become merely a post-graduate nursing specialty and still retain its distinct philosophy. The "nurse-midwife only" model is the easiest one to achieve legislatively. It poses few structural problems, since nurses already have a place in the medical system, and nursing schools already offer postgraduate obstetrical courses. For obvious reasons, the medical authorities view exclusive nurse-midwifery as the lesser of the midwifery evils. But is it the model that best serves consumers?

Nurses can make fine midwives. No question. Almost one third of our current practising midwives — nurses themselves — illustrate this amply. But the lay midwives provide countervailing proof that a fine midwife need not first be a nurse. A study of "Midwifery Outside the Nursing Profession," prepared at the University of Washington for state legislators, concluded that "midwives can be trained to render a high standard of services without having first undergone basic nursing education."[7] Internationally, midwifery and nursing are seen as two distinct professions.

It is unfortunately true that nursing in Canada remains largely the handmaiden of medicine. A radical front militates for independence with such roles as "nurse practitioner," but the success of their valiant struggle has been limited. Male doctors, having long depended on female nurses to cater to their needs, are generally unwilling to emancipate them. And many of the nursing institutions tend to reinforce the hierarchial status quo. A clear illustration is the case of two nurses practising midwifery in Ontario: Called in by the Ontario College of Nurses to discuss their activities, they were informed that their files had been passed along to the College of Physicians and Surgeons.[8] Clearly the higher authority!

Midwives trained in nursing schools to defer to doctors' authority would hardly serve the birthing public's best interests. Nurses should certainly have access to midwifery. But they must receive their training from midwives in a midwifery school, along with women of other backgrounds. Non-nurse-midwives must be allowed to balance the "medical" impact on midwifery training. Both the Midwives Alliance of North America and the prestigious International Confederation of Midwives support this position. Canadian nurse-midwives have recently been discovering that other midwives are more supportive of their political goals than is the nursing profession.

Parental input into the workings of a new midwifery profession is another essential safeguard. Any governing body, like the College of Midwives proposed in the 1984 Ontario Bill,[9] must be heavily weighted with consumers. These parents must be more than token appointees, rubber-stamping decisions about discipline and standards designed by midwives to suit their own professional interests. The consumers on the board must hold real power in order to protect parents' hard-won decision-making authority over their own births.

To further insure optimal service and client satisfaction, midwives should be allowed to practise in various settings and contexts. As well as employment in hospitals, doctors' offices, and (eventually) birthing centres, midwives might choose private practice with hospital privileges. Clients could then choose a particular midwife to suit their individual needs. She would provide care in the birthing venue of their choice, not merely come as part of an institutional care package deal.

Preservation of the home birth option is another essential safeguard for midwifery as we know it. More than just a service to a small percentage of radical parents, home birth sets a standard for natural, family-centred birth. It provides a balancing perspective to the hospital birth norms. Midwives who can operate with minimal technology in the intimate home setting carry that confidence and ambition into hospitals. They are less likely to catch the "birth terror" epidemic among high risk hospital practitioners today. Home birth midwives provide a check to creeping interventionism.

Particular communities will isolate other factors they wish to protect through the legislative process, but one final safeguard that must not be omitted is the "granny clause." Originally developed to allow elderly granny midwives to continue practising when new standards for midwifery were legislated, it can similarly protect our active new midwives. Without it, experienced midwives would be forced to undergo years of formal training to meet legal qualifications. For many mature women with families, financial responsibilities and clients to attend to, re-education would prove impossible. Under a granny clause, they need only to prove their competence to continue practising.

We cannot afford to banish the dedicated core group of practising midwives who developed the care model we so admire. We need them to guard the philosophy of the new midwifery, and illustrate its norms. Indeed, it would be absurd to take those midwives with the most up-to-date skills and experience out of circulation, just when we need to train a nation's worth of new midwives.

Models for Legalization

Each jurisdiction should assess for itself what model of legalization and regulation would provide optimal midwifery care. With a critical eye to legislative accomplishments and errors elsewhere, they can seek to embody the best of their own brand of midwifery, while correcting its shortcomings.

Writing briefs and legislation, some midwives are becoming veritable lay lawyers. They have learned to assess the subtle differences between regulating structures like licensing, registration and certification. They weigh options to decide what forms of legalization would best safeguard midwifery autonomy *and* client control. What is the public ready to accept? What models will seem feasible to the health authorities? Where is that wise compromise that will win legal, insured, universally accessible midwifery services within the decade, without undermining any basic principles?

Healthy debate rages within the midwifery movement. We read articles "Against the Licensing of Midwives"[10] and then the opposite. Experience in the political process can alter even the most concerted stance. The midwives' coalition preparing a brief for the Ontario Health Professions Legislative Review Committee was committed at the outset to a "buyer beware" concept of different kinds of midwives using "informed consent" with their clients. Political advisors convinced them that such a proposal would not be taken seriously by a government that sees its role as protecting the people. The midwives' coalition eventually arrived at an opposite stance, asking for exclusive right to practise and the protected title of Certified Midwife (C.M.).[11]

Beyond modes of regulation, there is the question of whether to have different kinds of midwives. Dr. Price describes a vision of interlocking roles for community-based lay midwives, nurse-midwives, obstetrical nurses, general practitioners and obstetricians. He assigns to the lay midwife the bulk of births, suggesting that 90% need her compassionate presence most. She need not have years of formal training, because she can call on the nurse-midwife, who has more technical expertise. Dr. Price separates the "compassionate" and "technical" roles, fearing that the union is unlikely in a mass profession of midwives. He does admit that current midwives with "the calling," manage to combine both.

Midwife Vicki van Wagner has examined such systems elsewhere. She believes it won't work in the long run, that any sub-categories within the profession will provoke a divide-and-conquer strategy from medical adversaries. Would a community-based midwife with less technical training than her nurse-midwife colleague be allowed to remain "in charge" of her normal birthing clients in hospital? Would her role be taken seriously by medical personnel? Van Wagner suggests that the community midwives would be rapidly disempowered.

The process of creating a working model for midwifery in our health care system is a difficult one. Different models will suit different jurisdictions. But in order that the midwifery system really work, all concerned parties must be involved in the development process. Doctors, nurses, hospital administrators and health bureaucrats must be invited to join midwives and consumers in their deliberations. Although concensus will be difficult to achieve, any unilateral decision that creates enduring opposition will not serve the public interest.

Changing Attitudes: Midwifery and Medicine

> Most of us have not grown up in a midwifery environment. . .once we see it working in an organized program, then doubts will disappear.
>
> — Dr. Ray Osborne,
> Obstetrician

Structural, legal and institutional change is not enough. The real triumph of the midwifery movement will be measured by changing attitudes. Especially among medical professionals, but also among the midwives and the public. New structures will not stand or serve without fundamental attitudinal changes. And these can only be brought about by communication and contact.

Doctors and nurses need to see first hand that midwifery will not just take away from their domains. It can add something new, provide different ways to do better work. Much of the medical prejudice against midwifery is born of ignorance and misinformation. Once doctors and nurses can meet midwives in a non-threatening environment and see what they actually do, prejudices will tend to dissolve. Dr. Price prophesies that: ''In the face of something working that they can't explain, doctors' preconceptions will go down the drain. The structures currently hampering doctors will collapse by evolution. Midwifery will change obstetrics and medicine. I've seen it happening.''

Once the oppressed/oppressor battle lines are dissolved, and midwives have access to the workings of hospitals, they will more readily appreciate the effectiveness of *appropriate* obstetrical technology, and the dedication of some doctors and nurses. Legalization will take a load off their shoulders by giving them clear access to medical support when a situation calls for it. Along with the load, the chip will also go.

And midwives will in turn take a load off doctors' shoulders. In 1989 we may well hear reiterated this revelation about a British doctor, published in the Canadian Medical Association Journal in 1929:

Since he obtained the assistance of two or three trained midwives, he reduced the incidence of his forceps deliveries from 30 percent to 3 percent, and. . .now had leisure for reading and attending society meetings, which he never had before.[12]

The lengthy process of achieving legalization provides opportunities to initiate dialogue and contact between midwives and medical people. In Alberta, it was a recommendation from the Health Occupations Board that brought the practising Domicilliary Midwives and the Western Nurse-Midwives together to form a united Midwifery Task Force. In Ontario, the Health Professions Review process called for bilateral meetings between the midwifery coalition and various medical, nursing and hospital organizations. Practising lay midwives actually sat down with the College of Physicians and Surgeons for the first time.[13]

"Creating Unity," the Midwives Alliance of North America conference in Toronto in November 1984 was another forum for contact between midwives, consumers, nurses and doctors. Medical professionals were invited to air their opinions and influence the actions of the midwifery movement.

Pilot projects like the New Grace Hospital midwifery program, from 1982 to 1984, are another vehicle for attitudinal change. Sacrificing their time on a volunteer basis, four midwives demonstrated the viability of their profession under the eye of hospital personnel. They also contributed medically acceptable statistical evidence favourable to midwifery.[14] Further midwifery pilot projects are now rumoured at two Ontario and one Alberta institution.

Perhaps the ideal forum for mutual understanding between midwifery and medicine is the birthing centre, that missing link in the Canadian maternity system. Like midwifery, the advent of birthing centres is now deemed inevitable. It will service growing public demand for an alternative birthing venue, but it will also present a clean-slate setting where doctors and midwives can observe each other. Perhaps attached to hospitals, but detached from historical prejudices, birthing centres may provide that "organized programme" doctors need to see working.

Some Benefits of our Midwifery-To-Be

All over the world there exists in every society a small group of women who feel themselves strongly attracted to give care to other women during pregnancy and childbirth. . . .Failure to make use of this rather small group of highly motivated people is regrettable, and a sin against the principle of subsidiarity.[15]
— Professor G.J. Kloosterman

The Canadian health care system has clearly sinned against midwives and the public. The result has been a style of maternity care that is most kindly described as "fragmented, uncoordinated and sometimes inadequate."[16] In atoning for the sin of excluding midwives, our governments will clearly be taking progressive steps. But just how far-reaching the social consequences of our new midwifery system might be, we are only beginning to discover.

Certainly there will be financial savings, safety improvements and increased consumer satisfaction. The benefits of continuous preventative care will accrue disproportionately to the disadvantaged population who need it most: Northern natives and Inuit, the inner-city poor, single and teenaged mothers. These groups may even escape their automatic high risk obstetrical status.

Women-centred midwifery care represents a significant advance in the struggle for feminist self-determination. Family-centred care offers some hope for that deeply threatened social unit. The respect for infant sensibilities inherent in midwifery bodes well for our children, and therefore the future. The effects of better births will eventually reach into every social and political realm.

The legalization of midwifery symbolizes a major evolutionary step in Canadian birth culture, and indeed in our culture and society at large. The birthing system we now militate to change was designed to meet the needs of another time, as Dr. Murray Enkin describes:

> The overriding need of our industrial society was for a labile, rapidly adaptive, mobile work force. One that would be available whenever the assembly line called it. A work force that would leave home freely, shedding no tears; that would wrench no bonds because there were no bonds to wrench. That would not feel uprooted because it had no roots. . .and so a system of birth practices were gradually built up that tended to blur, or even totally block, parental attachment. A system of birth practices which foster independence — and insecurity.[17]

In the context of our post-industrial society, our "information age" or "new age," assembly-line birth has become an anachronism. Enlightened parents and professionals describe it as an injustice and an insult, a disservice to the next generation. Rather than mobility and independence, the survival tools for our children appear to be personal security and creativity.

Midwifery is a new age re-creation, its birth model in keeping with the times. Taking the best of medicine along, midwifery adds impetus to the social evolution of the 1980s.

The popularization of midwifery is inevitable, because more and more parents will refuse to accept less. However, the timetable for achieving legalization depends largely on the power of public demand for political change.

Even cynical observers agree that accessible midwifery will become a reality in Canada over the next five to ten years. The midwives are prepared, the public is active and anxious, and governments are rapidly becoming convinced. As the medical profession begins to accept and even embrace a midwifery care option for Canadians, clearly the time has come. And as NAPSAC co-founder Lee Stewart once pronounced: "There is no idea so powerful as one whose time has come."

Notes

1. J. Cherry and J.C. Cameron, "Comparison of Hospital Charges Generated by Certified Nurse-Midwives and Physicians' Clients," *Journal of Nurse-Midwifery*, Jan, Feb. 1982, pp. 7-11.
   A. Dempkowski, "Future Prospects of Nurse-Midwifery In the United States," *Journal of Nurse-Midwifery*, March, April 1982, pp. 9-15.
2. RNABC, "Report of the Task Committee on the Future of Nurse-Midwives," June 1976, pp. 6-7.
3. "Report of the Joint Committee of the CHA, CMA and CNA on the Transfer of Functions Between Doctors and Nurses in the Hospital," Ottawa, June 1972.
4. A. Dempkowski, "Future Prospects of Nurse-Midwifery in the United States," *Journal of Nurse-Midwifery,* March, April 1982, pp. 9-15.
   J.A. Sullivan, R.N. et al, "Overcoming Barriers to the Employment and Utilization of the Nurse-Practitioner," *American Journal of Public Health,* Nov. 1978, pp. 1097-1103.
5. Elizabeth Davis quoted in *Issue*, Vol. 3, No. 2, Spring 1983, p. 2.
6. J.S. Tomkinson, "Professional Inter-relationship: The Midwife and the Physician," *International Journal of Gynaecology and Obstetrics,* 17:1979, pp. 99-101.
7. "Midwifery Outside the Nursing Profession," University of Washington, Seattle, 1980, p. 90.
8. "Nurse Midwives Reported," *Issue*, Vol. 1, No. 4, Winter 1981.
9. Bill 48, "An Act to Establish Midwifery as a Self-Governing Profession," Legislature of Ontario, First Reading, April 26, 1984.
10. J. Parvatti Baker, "Against The Licensing of Midwives," *Nurturing*, Winter 1984, pp. 103-106.
11. Vicki Van Wagner et al, "Brief on Midwifery Care in Ontario," Appendix A.
12. A.D.B. Editorial, "On Maternity Teaching and the Obstetric Nurse," *Canadian Medical Association Journal,* 1929, p. 647.
13. Vicki van Wagner, Meeting with the CPSO, Wednesday, April 18, 1984, Toronto.
14. Leslie Weatherson et al, "Statistics for the Low Risk Clinic, Grace Hospital," Vancouver, April 1984.
15. G.J. Kloosterman M.D., in *Midwifery Is A Labour of Love,* Maternal Health Society, Vancouver, April 1984, p. 8.
16. "Statement on the Nurse-Midwife," Canadian Nurses' Association, Ottawa, CNA 1974, Revised 1978.
17. Murray Enkin, M.D. quoted in "Birth: Impact on the Participants," D. Mandel, M.D., Unpublished Paper first presented at St. Michael's Hospital, Toronto, 1978.

Appendix A
How to Find a Midwife
(Or make contact with the midwifery community)

The concentrations of actively practising midwives vary from province to province. Some midwifery support organizations and professional organizations are more visible than others.

Through the following contacts, organizations and publications you should be able to find out if there is a practising midwife who can serve you.

By joining the organizations and subscribing to publications, you can help to bring midwives out of the closet, and promote legalization in your province. You will also find information about available birthing alternatives, and connect with like-minded parents.

These provincial organizations will link enquirers up with any local chapters or associations.

British Columbia

There are approximately 40 practising midwives and apprentices, concentrated in Victoria, Vancouver and the Nelson area.

MTF B.C.
(The Interdisciplinary Midwifery Task Force of British Columbia)
926 School Green
Vancouver, B.C. V6H 3N7
Gale Gray (604) 738-9601

A consumer organization with political goals.

MABC
(The Midwives Association of British Columbia)
P.O. Box 46698, Station "G"
Vancouver, B.C. V6R 4K8

A professional association for practising and non-practising midwives of all backgrounds.

Maternal Health News
P.O. Box 46563, Station "G"
Vancouver, B.C. V6R 4G8
Midwifery Editor: Debbie Farnsworth

A publication that serves the midwifery and birth communities. Subscription included in MTF membership.

Alberta

There are approximately ten practising midwives and apprentices, concentrated in Calgary and Edmonton.

CAPSAC

(Calgary Association of Parents & Professionals for Safe Alternatives in Childbirth)
1123-10th Street S.E.
Calgary, Alberta T6G 3E3
Catherine Reid (403) 272-7393

A consumer organization for the Calgary area.

ASAC

(Association for Safe Alternatives in Childbirth)
Box 1197
Main Post Office
Edmonton, Alberta T5J 2M4
Rebecca Das (403) 437-0187

A consumer organization for the Edmonton area.

ACRDMA

(Alberta Council and Register of Domicilliary Midwives Association)
507 Tavender Rd. N.W.
Calgary, Alberta T2K 3M3
Sandra Botting, President (403) 275-3997

or

217 Farrell Properties
52307 RG Rd. 213
Sherwood Park, Alberta T8G 1C1
Noreen Walker, Vice-President

A professional organization of practising domicilliary midwives.

WNMA

(Western Nurse-Midwives Association)
25 52252 Range Rd. 215
Sherwood Park, Alberta T8E 1B7
Joyce Ralyea, President

A professional organization of practising and non-practising midwives with nursing backgrounds.

Alberta MTF
(The Alberta Midwifery Task Force)
c/o Sandra Botting
507 Tavender Rd. N.W.
Calgary, Alberta
T2K 3M3

A newly-formed political organization unifying ACRDMA and WNMA interests in legalization.

Birth Issues
Calgary Editor
Stan Hingston (403) 270-4196
c/o CAPSAC

or

Edmonton Editor
Henriette Douzier (403) 487-5532
c/o ASAC

A province-wide publication that serves the alternative birthing community. Subscription included in CAPSAC or ASAC membership.

Saskatchewan

There are 2 practising midwives in the Regina area. (Four others have also been active until recently.)

SASAC
(Saskatchewan Association for Safe Alternatives in Childbirth)
2071 Montague Street
Regina, Saskatchewan S4T 3J8
Donna Burton, President (306) 522-6325

An organization of midwives and consumers.

SASAC News
P.O. Box 3301
Nipawin, Saskatchewan S0E 1E0
Barbara Scriver, Editor

A publication serving the alternative birthing community in the province. Subscription included in SASAC membership.

Manitoba

There are three practising midwives and apprentices in the Winnipeg district. There is, as yet, no midwifery organization or newsletter, but enquiries can be made to:

Darlene Birch
General Delivery
St. Eustache, Manitoba R0H 1H0

Ontario

There are approximately 30 practising midwives and apprentices, concentrated in Toronto, Ottawa, the Kitchener-Waterloo and Thunder Bay areas.

MTF Ontario
(The Midwifery Task Force of Ontario)
P.O. Box 489, Station T
Toronto, Ontario M6B 4C2
Co-ordinators: Holly Nimmons (416) 537-2257
Arlene Thorn (416) 294-4832

A consumer organization with political goals.

The Association of Ontario Midwives
P.O. Box 85, Station C
Toronto, Ontario M6J 3M7
Contact: Merryn Tate (416) 652-1521
Rena Porteous (416) 336-2488

A professional organization of midwives of all backgrounds, formerly the Ontario Association of Midwives (OAM) and the Ontario Nurse-Midwives Association (ONMA).

Issue
c/o Theo Dawson, Editor
General Delivery
Locust Hill, Ontario L0H 1J0

A newsletter serving midwifery supporters. Subscription included with MTF Ontario membership.

The Ontario Midwife
c/o Association of Ontario Midwives
Editor: Heather Simopoulos

A newsletter of practical interest to active midwives.

Quebec

There are approximately 20 practising midwives and apprentices, concentrated in the Montreal area.

Naissance-Renaissance
C.P. 249, Station E
Montreal, P.Q. H2T 3A7
Contact: Diane Eire (514) 845-3368

An organization of midwives and consumers promoting midwifery and birth alternatives.

L'Une à l'Autre
c/o Naissance Renaissance
Editor: Hélène Cornellier

A magazine serving the birthing community.

New Brunswick

One midwife has been practising in the Moncton area in recent years. There is no midwifery organization, but those interested might contact:

Anne-Marie Arsenault
92 Portledge Avenue
Moncton, N.B. E1C 5S7

Nova Scotia

Three midwives and apprentices have been practising in the Halifax area.

APSAC Nova Scotia
(Association of Parents & Professionals for Safe Alternatives in Childbirth of Nova Scotia)
P.O. Box 67
Armdale, N.S. B3L 4J7
Contact: Valerie O'Day
(902) 479-2969

A consumer organization. Membership includes the APSAC Newsletter.

Midwifery Coalition of Nova Scotia
c/o Holly Bell
6316 Willow Street
Halifax, N.S. B3L 1N9
(902) 423-2086

An organization aimed at legalization and public education, formed in 1984.

Prince Edward Island

There are approximately seven midwives and apprentices practising.

P.E.I. Holistic Childbirth Association
c/o Arlene Arsenault
R.R. #1, Montague, P.E.I. C0A 1R0
(902) 892-3730
(902) 962-2275

An organization of midwives and consumers.

Newfoundland

A few midwives practise legally in the health care system in Newfoundland and Labrador. No independent midwives are known to be active, outside of native or Inuit communities in Labrador.

There is no organization to promote midwifery, but there is an official midwifery training program at Memorial University of Newfoundland.

Those interested might contact:

Hope Toumishey
Assistant Professor
School of Nursing
Memorial University
St. John's, Newfoundland A1C 5S7

Yukon and North-West Territories

Practising midwives have not yet been identified. No midwifery support organizations or publications are known. Interested midwives and consumers should contact:

Midwives Association of Canada
251 West 20th Ave.
Vancouver, B.C. V5Y 2C5
Coordinator: Lee Saxell

A bilingual national organization formed in 1984 to act as a liaison between midwifery organizations across Canada, and to assist in forming new groups.

If there is no organization supporting midwifery and birth alternatives in your area, contact the **Midwives Association of Canada** to find out how you could start one.

United States

MANA
Midwives' Alliance of North America
P.O. Box 11171
Bainbridge Island, Washington 98110

NAPSAC International
P.O. Box 267
Marble Hill, Missouri 63764

These international organizations will direct those interested to national, state and local professional and consumer associations concerned with midwifery.

Appendix B
How to Choose a Midwife

There is no foolproof method for choosing the right midwife. In fact, many parents have no choice at all. But if you do have more than one midwife around, or you're weighing the midwife option against a doctor, the following list of 22 leading questions may help.

You don't need to ask them all. (If you do, she may begin to wonder if this is an inquisition.) You will have other personal and specific questions to add. For example, medical conditions or maternity factors in your family. Detailed answers to two or three questions may satisfy.

Talk with more than one midwife, and many other mothers. Comparison shopping is kosher. Use these questions to cue your own curiosity. Research with your intellect and then go with your instincts.

1. Why are you a midwife?

Listen for personal motivations that suggest a balance of ego attachment to the midwife role with a genuine service orientation. Be wary of those who condemn the whole health care delivery system or are simply captured by the romance of birth.

2. What have your personal birth experiences been like?

Most midwives are mothers. Their assessments of their own birthing histories, good or bad, will reveal a lot about what they have to offer — and why.

3. How did you become a midwife?

Has this person seized every training opportunity open to her? How long did she study/apprentice? With whom? Is she trained to work in the home birth setting? Is her training up-to-date and her experience current?

4. How many births have you attended?

At home? In hospital? As an apprentice/observer or as a primary caregiver? Proposed standards suggest that a qualified midwife should have been at 50 labours and births. In rural settings, however, this volume could take years to accumulate. How does her experience compare with other midwives in the area?

5. What complications have you handled?

Has she at least seen all the major complications competently managed? For example, maternal hemorrhage and fetal distress? Has she coped with neonatal death?

6. Do you have any statistics you could show?

Most midwives do not have a big enough birth base to be statistically significant. But a summary of the outcomes of her births could be very useful if you've researched enough to interpret it. It would reveal any tendency toward interventionism.

7. What is your hospital transfer rate for planned home births?

Some midwives are cautious and frequently transport. Others rarely transport for any reason short of medical emergency. The norm is 10% to 15% transfer for first-time mothers, the majority of these for simple failure to progress. Do you feel comfortable with her reasons and attitudes toward hospital transfer? Will she stay with you in hospital?

8. Describe your role at a home birth. At hospital birth?

Does her perception of her role match your perception of your needs?

9. What is your relationship with local doctors and hospitals?

Has she developed trust or at least grudging respect from some medical professionals? Can she offer adequate medical back-up if you need it? Is she welcome in hospital? Is she working on it?

10. What equipment do you carry and what procedures do you follow?

Many midwives now carry oxygen, infant resuscitation equipment and anti-hemorrhage drugs. Does she regularly check fetal heart tones, maternal blood pressure, urine, etc. Be sure she is competent to attend to your basic medical needs, prenatally, through labour and delivery, and the postpartum.

11. Who is eligible for a home birth with you?

What are her risk-screening factors? Do you qualify? Are her safety standards high enough to make you a comfortable home birth candidate? Would she tell you if you are better off in hospital?

12. Are you prepared to take full responsibility as the primary caregiver?

Beware of "labour coaches" who are not midwives. They offer valuable services but are not trained adequately to take responsibility for birth outcomes. Your midwife should be competent to handle a whole normal birth, along with you. Without a doctor actively participating.

13. Do you provide continuous care?

How much time will this midwife spend with you, and will she be available consistently through your childbearing cycle? What is her schedule for prenatal visits? The norm is once a month for 30 minutes to an hour, working up to weekly visits in the final month. Postpartum visits are also essential for both home and hospital birthing. Three to five is the average number, depending on need and distance.

14. How many births do you attend per month?

A high average will assure you lots of current experience and skills. A low average — one or two births a month — may mean more individual time. Which serves your needs best?

15. Who is your back-up midwife?

Someone should be available to provide care if your midwife isn't. You should arrange to meet her. Ideally, midwives do not work in isolation. They need each other, and you may need a second midwife.

16. Will we have an equal partnership in responsibility?

Does she respect your rights to make your own birthing decisions with her expert advice? Is she liable to "take over" or to "opt out"? Is she comfortable with all your questions? And you with the honesty of her answers?

17. What is your political and legal position as a midwife?

Is she frank about her legal status? What expectations does she have of you in any politically difficult situation? Will you sign an informed consent indicating each of your responsibilities and abilities?

18. How do you keep up your skills?

Is she attending workshops and conferences? Reading new birthing literature? Involved in peer review rounds with other midwives? Midwifery is a developing art and science. She needs to find some way to keep up with new developments. Obviously, opportunities will vary from place to place.

19. What are your particular strengths and weaknesses as a midwife?

Candid answers are important. Every midwife ought to recognize her own weaknesses. Ideally, she has found a partner/partners with corresponding strengths. Nobody is perfect. But is she trying to get better all the time?

20. What do you consider "normal"?

Does her "range of normal" give you enough time and scope to follow your own birthing process? Is she tied to medical timetables, or just concerned that mother and baby remain healthy and cope well?

21. What do you charge? Why?

Be sure to agree on fees and a payment schedule. Feel free to ask how she calculates her fees (according to hours, supply costs, equipment expenses, etc.). If you genuinely need a lower fee, ask if she has a sliding scale geared to income. Do be prepared to pay.

22. How do you feel about working with me/us?

Does she have any reservations about working with you: medical, practical or personality factors?

Then ask yourself: How do I/we feel about working with her?

Do you trust her skills? Do you like her? Can you rely on her? Think about it for a few days. Discuss her with your partner. Interview other midwives. Ask other clients. Give credence to your instincts. Then decide.

If you have given the question your full attention, be confident that no one else knows better. Choose your midwife. Indulge yourself in her care.

Bibliography

Books

Abbott, Maude. *A History of Medicine in the Province of Quebec*. Toronto: Macmillan, 1931.

Arms, Suzanne. *A Season to be Born*. New York: Harper Colophon, 1973.

_____. *Immaculate Deception*. New York: Bantam, 1979.

Baldwin, Rahima. *Special Delivery*. Millbrae, California: Les Femmes Publishing, 1979.

Brennan, Barbara and Joan Rattner Heilman. *The Complete Book of Midwifery*. New York: E.P. Dutton, 1977.

Brooks, Tanya and Linda Bennett. *Giving Birth at Home*. Curritos, California: ACHI, 1976.

Buss, Fran Leeper. *La Partera*. Toronto: John Wiley and Sons, 1980.

Chard, T. and M. Richards eds. *The Benefits and Hazards of the New Obstetrics*. London: Heinemann, 1977.

Cohen, N.W. and L.J. Estner. *Silent Knife: Cesarean Prevention and Vaginal Birth After Cesarean*. South Hadley, Mass.: Bergin and Garvey Publishers Inc., 1983.

Courter, Gay. *The Midwife*. New York: New American Library, 1981. (Fiction.)

Davis, Elizabeth. *A Guide To Midwifery: Heart and Hands*. New Mexico: John Muir Publishing, 1981.

Donnison, Jean. *Midwives and Medical Men*. London: Heinemann, 1977.

Ehrenreich, Barbara and Dierdre English. *For Her Own Good*. New York: Doubleday, 1979.

_____. *Complaints and Disorders: The Sexual Politics of Sickness*. New York: Feminist Press, 1973.

_____. *Witches, Midwives and Nurses: A History of Women Healers*. New York: Feminist Press, 1983.

Elkins, Valmai. *The Rights of the Pregnant Parent*. Toronto: Waxwing Press, 1976.

_____. *Birth Report*. Toronto: Lester and Orpin Dennys, 1983.

Eloesser, Leo et al. *Pregnancy, Childbirth and the Newborn*. Instituto Indigenista Interamericano, 1973.

Gaskin, Ina May. *Spiritual Midwifery*. Summertown, Tennessee: The Book Publishing Co., 1980.

Hazell, L.D. *Birth Goes Home*. Scarborough: Catalyst Publishing Co., 1974.

_____. *Commonsense Childbirth*. New York: Berkely Books, 1980.

Howell, W.B. *F.J. Shepherd - Surgeon: His Life and His Times*. Toronto: J. Dent and Sons, 1934.

Johnson, Ingrid and Paul Johnson. *The Paper Midwife*. Dunedin, New Zealand: Caveman Press, 1980.

Kitzinger, Sheila. *Birth at Home*. New York: Penguin, 1979.

_____. *The Complete Book of Pregnancy and Childbirth*. New York: Knopf, 1981.

_____, and J.A. Davies eds. *The Place of Birth*. Oxford: Oxford Medical Publications, 1978.

Lang, Raven. *Birth Book*. Ben Lomond, California: Genesis Press, 1972.

Leboyer, Frederick. *Birth Without Violence.* New York: Knopf, 1975.

Litoff, Judy B. *American Midwives: 1860 To The Present.* London: Greenwood Press, 1978.

Lumley, Judith and Jill Astbury. *Birth Rites, Birth Rights.* Australia: Sphere Books, 1980.

Miles, Margaret F. *Textbook For Midwives.* Edinburgh: Churchill Livingstone, 1975.

Peterson, Gayle. *Birthing Normally.* Berkeley, California: Mindbody Press, 1981.

Romalis, Shelley. *Childbirth Alternatives to Medical Control.* Austin: University of Texas Press, 1981.

Rothman, Barbara Katz. *In Labor: Women and Power in the Birthplace.* New York: W.W. Norton and Co., 1982.

Sousa, Marion. *Childbirth At Home.* New York: Bantam, 1977.

Stewart, David. *The Five Standards for Safe Childbearing.* Marble Hill, Mo.: NAPSAC Reproductions, 1981.

————————————, and Lee Stewart eds. *21st Century Obstetrics Now!* Volumes I and II. Chapel Hill, Mo.: NAPSAC Reproductions 1977.

————————————————————. *Compulsory Hospitalization: Freedom of Choice In Childbirth?* Volumes I, II, and III. Marble Hill, Mo.: NAPSAC Reproductions, 1979.

Verny, Thomas and John Kelly. *The Secret Life of the Unborn Child.* New York: Delta Books, 1981.

Weir, G.M. *Survey of Nursing Education In Canada.* Toronto: University of Toronto Press, 1932.

Child at Risk. Senate Committee Report. Ottawa: Supply and Services Canada, 1980.

Maternity Care in the World. Second Edition. International Federation of Gynaecology and Obstetrics/International Confederation of Midwives, 1976.

Midwifery is a Labour of Love. Vancouver: Maternal Health Society, 1981.

National Council of Women Yearbook. 1932.

Periodical Articles

Anderson, S.F. "Childbirth as a Pathological Process: An American Perspective." *American Journal of Maternal and Child Health.* Vol. 2, 1977.

Antler, Joyce and D.M. Fox. "The Movement Towards a Safe Maternity Care." *Bulletin of the History of Medicine.* 1976.

Bernstein, Hannah. "Study Urged Into Status of Unborn Child." *Canadian Bar Foundation News.* Vol. 2, No. 3, March 1984.

Biggs, C.L. "The Case of the Missing Midwives." *Ontario History.* LXXV, No. 1, March 1983.

Botting, Sandra. "News Update." *Birth Issues.* Vol. 1, No. 1, Nov./Dec. 1983.

Caldero-Barcia, R. "Some Consequences of Obstetrical Interference." *Birth and the Family Journal.* Vol. 2, No. 2.

Cherry, J. and J.C. Cameron. "Comparison of Hospital Charges Generated by Certified Nurse-Midwives' and Physicians' Clients." *Journal of Nurse-Midwifery.* Vol. 27, No. 1, Jan./Feb. 1982.

Dempkowski, A. "Future Prospects of Nurse-Midwifery in the United States." *Journal of Nurse-Midwifery.* Vol. 27, No. 2, Mar./Apr. 1982.

Devitt, Neil. "The Transition From Home to Hospital Birth in the U.S. 1930-1960." *Birth and the Family Journal.* Summer 1977.

Fitzgerald, Linda. "Home Birth: An Alternative on Trial." *New Age.* Vol. 6, No. 6, Dec. 1980.

Gaskin, Ina May. *The Practising Midwife.* No. 11, Fall 1980.

Haverkamp, A. et al. "The Evaluation of Continuous Fetal Heart Rate Monitoring in High Risk Pregnancy." *American Journal of Obstetrics and Gynaecology.* Vol. 125, 1976.

Hopkinson, Blaise. "Inquest on Baby Death." *Toronto Sun.* July 15, 1982.

Kieran, Michael. "Proposal to License Midwives." *The Globe and Mail.* June 25, 1982.

Landsberg, Michele. "You Wrote Reams About Midwives." *The Toronto Star.* April 21, 1983.

Meere, Vil. "Pros and Cons of Home Birth." *Medical Post.* July 27, 1980.

Mehl, Lewis E. et al. "Outcomes of Elective Home Births." *Journal of Reproductive Medicine.* Vol. 19, No. 5, November 1977.

_____. "Evaluation of Outcomes of Non-Nurse Midwives." *Women and Health.* Vol. 5, No. 2, Summer 1980.

O'Day, V. and R. O'Day. *APSAC Nova Scotia Newsletter.* No. 2, February 1984.

Oppenheimer, J. "Childbirth in Ontario: The Transition from Home to Hospital in the Early Twentieth Century." *Ontario History.* Vol. LXXV, No. 1, March 1983.

Parvatti, Baker, J. "Against the Licensing of Midwives." *Nurturing.* Winter 1984.

Pearse, W.H. Editorial. *ACOG Newsletter.* July 1977.

Phaire, J.T. and A.H. Sellers. "A Study of Maternal Deaths in the Province of Ontario." *Canadian Journal of Public Health.* Vol. 25, December 1934.

Sosa, Roberto et al. "The Effect of a Supportive Companion on Perinatal Problems, Length of Labor, and Mother-Infant Interaction." *New England Journal of Medicine.* Vol. 303, No. 11, September 11, 1980.

Stratmeyer, M.E. "Research in Ultrasound Bioeffects." *Birth and the Family Journal.* Vol. 7, No. 2, Summer 1980.

Sullivan, J.A. et al. "Overcoming Barriers to the Employment and Utilization of the Nurse-Practitioner." *American Journal of Public Health.* Vol. 68, No. 11, November 1978.

Tait, Mark. "M.D.s to Battle Bid Allowing Midwives." *Calgary Herald.* October 28, 1982.

Tolagsen, S. *Genesis.* Vancouver, May 1980.

Tomkinson, J.S. "Professional Interrelationship: The Midwife and the Physician." *International Journal of Gynaecology and Obstetrics.* Vol. 17, 1979.

Vosu, Ava. *Issue.* Vol. 2, No. 2, Summer 1982.

Wright, Gerald. "Midwives Maligned." *The Kitchener-Waterloo Record.* June 30, 1983.

Editorial. "On Maternity Teaching and the Obstetrical Nurse." *Canadian Medical Association Journal.* 1929.

Editorial. "Meddlesome Midwifery." *Canada Lancet.* Vol 17, 1885.

Editorial. *The Globe and Mail.* August 24, 1885.

Editorial. "Midwifery on Trial." *NAPSAC News.* Vol. 7, No. 3, Fall 1982.

Editorial. "Midwifery in Transition." *NAPSAC News.* Vol. 8, No. 2, Summer 1983.

Editorial. "Midwife Father Fined in Scotland." *The Practising Midwife.* Winter 1981.

Reports, Briefs, Statistics, Unpublished Papers, Legal Proceedings

Anderson, Cheryl et al. "Birth Statistics. Vancouver Free Childbirth Education Centre." Unpublished. February 1973 — February 1974.

Armstrong, Janice. "The Risks and Benefits of Home Birth." Toronto. Unpublished. 1982.

Barrington, Eleanor. "Legalization of Midwifery." Brief to National Action Committee on the Status of Women. January 1984.

Begin, Monique. *Hansard 2583.* March 29, 1984.

Burton-Fripp, Carol, Producer. "Medical Intervention in Childbirth." *Speaking Out* series. T.V. Ontario. First aired November 10, 1983.

Cayley, David. "The Medicalization of Childbirth." *Morningside.* CBC Radio. Fall 1981.

Haire, Doris. "The Cultural Warping of Childbirth." A Special Report. International Childbirth Education Association. 1972.

Hodnett, E.D. "The Effects of Person-Environment Interactions on Selected Childbirth Outcomes of Women Having Home and Hospital Births." Doctoral Thesis. University of Toronto, 1983.

Malloch, Leslie. "Indian Health: Indian Medicine." Unpublished paper for Union of Ontario Indians. Toronto, 1982.

Mandel, D. "Birth: Impact on the Participants." Unpublished paper presented at St. Michael's Hospital. Toronto, 1978.

Pullen, Sandra et al. "Statistics on Home Birth Midwifery Practice". December 1980 - December 1983. Edmonton, 1984.

Toane, Benjamin et al. "A Presentation to the College of Physicians and Surgeons." ASAC/CAPSAC. Edmonton, April 30, 1981.

van Wagner, Vicki. "The New Midwifery." Unpublished paper. Toronto, 1981.

_____ et al. "Midwives Coalition Brief to the Health Professions Legislative Review Committee." First Submission December 1983. Second Submission June 1984.

Weatherston, Leslie et al. "Statistics for the Low Risk Clinic, Grace Hospital." Vancouver, April 1984.

Wittmann, B.K. et al. "Hospital-Based Midwifery Care — Preliminary Results." Presented at the Annual General Meeting of the Society of Obstetricians and Gynaecologists of Canada. Vancouver, June 1983.

No Authors

"Act to Regulate the Qualifications of Practitioner of Medicine and Surgery in Upper Canada." Ch. 32, 29. Victoria, September 18, 1865.

"Amendment to the New Canada Health Act." Clauses 2 and 9. March 20, 1984.

Bill 48. "An Act to Establish Midwifery as a Self-Governing Profession." Legislature of Ontario. First Reading: April 26, 1984.

"Canadian Charter of Rights and Freedoms Challenge to the College of Physicians and Surgeons Resolution." Alberta Civil Liberties Association.

"Creating Unity." Second Annual Convention of the Midwives Alliance of North America. Toronto, October 31 — November 4, 1984.

"Depuis Que le Monde at Monde." Film. Produced by Naissance Renaissance. Montreal, 1981.

"Home Birth Information and Data Gathering Survey." Health and Welfare Canada Project No. 1216-9-144. Nelson, B.C.

"Midwifery Law." *Childbearing Families and the Law Series*. Community Task Force on Maternal and Child Health. Health and Welfare Canada Project 1216-6-132. Winnipeg.

"Midwifery Outside the Nursing Profession." Report to the State Legislature Prepared by the University of Washington. Seattle, 1980.

"Number and Percentage of Births Occurring in Hospital 1921-1973." Dominion Bureau of Statistics.

"Out of Hospital Births." Position Statement of the College of Physicians and Surgeons of Ontario. February 1983.

R.V. Carpenter et al. Preliminary Hearing. October 25, 26 and November 25, 1983. Halifax. Unreported.

R.V. Marsh. 1980. Victoria, B.C. Unreported.

"Report of the Joint Committee of the CHA, CMA and CNA on the Transfer of Functions Between Doctors and Nurses in the Hospital." Ottawa, June 1972.

"Report of the Task Committee on the Future of Nurse-Midwives." RNABC. June 1976.

Resolution 15 of the National Action Committee on the Status of Women. Annual General Meeting. March 18, 1984.

"Resolution Prohibiting Elective Domiciliary Midwifery by a Member." College of Physicians and Surgeons of Alberta. 1981.

Ritz, Jean. Inquest into the Death of . . . May 20, 21 and June 18, 1982. Kitchener. Coroner Jack Burger. Chief Coroner's Office of Ontario.

"Statement on the Nurse-Midwife." Canadian Nurses' Association. Ottawa, 1974. Revised 1978.

Steell, Simon Peter. Inquest into the Death of . . . July 12, 13, 14, 1982. Toronto. Coroner P. Tepperman. Chief Coroner's Office of Ontario.

Acknowledgements and Thanks

To my beloved husband, Steven Bush, for his boundless generosity and enduring emotional support.

To my midwives Theo Dawson and Mary Sharpe, for making midwifery care an intimate reality for me this past year.

To Dr. Nancy Harris and Dr. Kasari for supporting our birthing choices.

To the parents who honoured me with invitations to attend their births.

To all the midwives, parents, and children who unguardedly shared their experiences and emotions.

To the doctors who dared to be frank.

Thanks to the photographers, especially Bonnie Johnson of Ottawa, Mark Laforet of Vancouver and Bill Usher of Toronto. Their art adds volumes to my words. To Lesley Biggs and Jutta Mason for sharing their historical research. To all those who took me into their homes during my research travels.

Warm hugs to Theo, Mary, Holly Nimmons and Diane Kolida for reminding me that my work was important at moments when I lost courage. Diane enthusiastically typed the whole manuscript to meet my nervous deadlines.

Special appreciation to Caroline Walker and NC Press, for seeing that the time for a Canadian midwifery book has come. And to the Canada Council Explorations Program and the Ontario Arts Council for financial support.

Finally, to my Liam who inspired the writing of this book from in utero, and waited for it to be finished to be born.

To each and all of you who have contributed, whether or not your names appear in the text, my thanks for making this book truly a labour of love.

Eleanor Barrington,
Toronto,
November 1984